SOMEONE ELSE'S FACE IN THE MIRROR

SOMEONE ELSE'S FACE IN THE MIRROR

Identity and the New Science of Face Transplants

Carla Bluhm and Nathan Clendenin

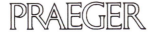

Westport, Connecticut
London

Library of Congress Cataloging-in-Publication Data

Bluhm, Carla, 1961–
    Someone else's face in the mirror : identity and the new
science of face transplants / by Carla Bluhm and Nathan Clendenin.
        p. cm.
    Includes bibliographical references and index.
    ISBN 978-0-313-35616-2 (alk. paper)
    1. Face—Transplantation. I. Clendenin, Nathan, 1984– II. Title.
    RD523.B55   2009
    617.5′20592—dc22   2008046769

British Library Cataloguing in Publication Data is available.

Library of Congress Catalog Card Number: 2008046769
ISBN: 978-0-313-35616-2

First published in 2009

Praeger Publishers, 88 Post Road West, Westport, CT 06881
An imprint of Greenwood Publishing Group, Inc.
www.praeger.com

Printed in the United States of America

The paper used in this book complies with the
Permanent Paper Standard issued by the National
Information Standards Organization (Z39.48-1984).

10   9   8   7   6   5   4   3   2   1

Contents

Acknowledgments

The endeavor of this collaborative project was made possible through the gracious support, encouragement, and interest provided by a number of people. We would like to especially thank John Broughton for being a compelling friend and challenging interlocutor, Michael Eigen for encouraging the work from its nascent days, Bohdan Pomahac for his generous offers to meet and discuss his work and share ideas, Susan Opotow for her keen eye and encouragement to turn the idea into a book, Andrew Kirby's editing suggestions, and Allen Furr for early conversations on the topic. Drs. Jean-Michel Dubernard, Bernard Devauchelle, and Laurent Lantieri graciously answered our questions and provided valuable information. Artists Daniel Lee and Paddy Hartley generously supplied images for the book.

We are grateful to many people at Allegheny College. We wish to specifically thank Dean Linda DeMeritt and the Academic Support Committee for providing encouragement and financial assistance. Many thanks go to the Psychology Department especially Cindy Hoesch who excelled in secretarial help and friendship and freshman seminar students for exploring and discussing face transplantation. The enthusiasm of so many Allegheny students has been wonderful. Erinn Alonso-Hohmann offered us tremendous research help and insight and Barb Steadman continues to provide enthusiasm and promotion.

Several people provided valuable specialized assistance for the book. Amy Ball guided us through the index and Alexandra Julio translated foreign languages. Katherine Grier at Cadmus kept the book on a timely track. Our editor at Praeger Debbie Carvalko has been really terrific. Thank you for finding us at APA and supporting our thoughts and ambitions to create a book on the topic of face transplantation.

Nathan would like to offer his personal appreciation to Glenn Holland, Suzanne Barnard, Mark Fratoni, Reena Sheth, Jessica Callanan, as well as friends from Allegheny College, Shimer College, and elsewhere. I would like to thank Carla Bluhm for sharing the opportunity to collaborate on this project with me, and for the careful attention that she has poured into this book since its infancy. I am extremely grateful to Henry, Veronica, and Frank Yocco; their kindness has been most helpful along the way. A lifetime of support from my parents, John and Dona Clendenin, and my brother Evan, has been especially important to me while completing this book. Thank you for always believing in me. Finally, I extend a special thank you to Norma Ann Yocco for the endless and encouraging love that she offered me throughout the writing of this book.

Carla would like to extend a personal thank you to Julie Patterson, Joshua and Stephanie Corrette-Bennett, Wayne Bissell, Mark Goral, Michael Nard, David Ball, George Endrizzi, Kathy Wildauer, and Sarah Conklin. I would like to thank my co-author Nathan Clendenin, who was first an excellent Allegheny student and then an excellent book writing partner. My extended family has been excited and supportive making the writing of the book even more meaningful. I am very thankful to all of them especially my parents Alvan and Barbara Bluhm, Adrienne and Mark Connelly, and Aaron, Adam, and Mercedes Bluhm. Bakhtin my kitty kept me nice company while I was writing. I am most grateful to my husband John Robertson for sharing his insight and ideas and providing support. My daughter Beryl was the most important driving force for me during the research and writing process. I could not have possibly written the book without her patience and love.

Introduction

On November 27, 2005, surgeons in France performed the world's first partial face transplant on a thirty-eight-year-old French woman named Isabelle Dinoire. She had suffered from a facial disfiguration created when her dog pawed off portions of her face while she slept in a drug-induced state of unconsciousness. Despite a culture well accustomed to the idea of pushing the human body beyond unheard of limits, the fact that, for the first time in human history, the face of one person had been successfully grafted onto another's head seemed to cause quite a stir of disbelief. Disbelief in spite of the fact that even as late as two weeks before Dinoire's procedure, a controversial episode of the FX television show *Nip/Tuck* titled "Hannah Tedesco" aired. In the program a young girl, badly disfigured on a carnival ride, received a full face transplant. The fact that such a procedure would be attempted in reality was so bold it left an alarming feeling in anyone coming across the news. From tabloid news sources to a prime-time interview with Barbara Walters, Dinoire seemed simultaneously to captivate and shock whatever audience that came across her. These responses signaled ambivalence in popular consciousness toward face transplants. Face transplants, or facial allograft procedures, have only been the punctuation to a string of bizarre transplant operations in recent years. Included here are successful hand and penis transplants—both of which had equally strange endings. The two recipients later had the organs removed at their own request and not as a result of issues of tissue rejection. In both cases, the psychological reality of facing each day with the hand or genitals of another person became alienating and ultimately unbearable for them.

Consider waking up each day unable to ignore the foreign body part sutured onto what was once a familiar region of your body. As difficult as it must be adjusting to the idea of possessing the internal organs of an alien body, now one must deal with the visual reality of possessing such an organ. What then of face transplants? Imagine the face, perhaps the most symbolically harried and clearest visible indicator of one's identity. Even in a disfigured form, it has now been erased, replaced with the face of another. A foreign visage, which once had a life of its own, the extreme nature of the procedure, which can be perceived as an excessive surgical intervention into a problem of identity has provoked a negative reaction even from an organization that works with likely candidates for face transplants. Yet, despite a seeming ambivalence toward face transplants, many people in the medical community seem hopeful about the possibilities that face transplantation may offer for those who suffer from severe facial disfigurement. Recent public relations campaigns undertaken by the hospitals wanting to perform face transplants have been appealing to this very hope. In a recent *Boston Globe* article, John Barker, a surgeon at the University of Louisville Medical Center and one of the researchers on their face transplant team said, "We have some patients with 120 [reconstructive] operations and you still look at them and it's hard to sit in front of them." Baker continued, "Think of exchanging that for one major surgery and maybe two or three others, and you look in the mirror and you look like a human being."[1] Such surgery may offer a humanizing dignity, an attention to a patient's sense of subjectivity. This attention has converted many in the medical world to its cause, despite concerns about medical ethics.

It is on account of this dignifying hope that face transplant procedures did not simply stop with Isabelle Dinoire. Rather than a one-off science-fiction urban legend, partial facial transplants have been performed three times since Dinoire's procedure. As many eagerly awaited the first face transplant procedure in America, two American hospitals raced to perform the procedure first. In July 2007, the Harvard University–affiliated Brigham and Women's Hospital in Boston, Massachusetts, announced that they had received ethics board permission to perform partial face transplantation on patients who have already been receiving immunosuppressant drug therapy.[2] Along with a surgical team at the Cleveland Clinic, the one at Brigham became the second surgical team in the United States to receive ethics committee approval to perform face transplants. Indeed, the aspirations of the team at the Cleveland Clinic were not simply to perform a partial facial allograft, but to perform the world's first full facial allograft procedure. In

December 2008, Dr. Maria Siemionow led a transplant team at the Cleveland Clinic in completing the first face transplant to be performed in America. In addition to being America's first, the procedure was one of the first of the world's nearly full face transplants, as the procedure consisted of transplanting more than just lower portions of the face, but also upper palette and teeth. As opposed to a partial allograft, which in Dinoire's case entailed the dermatological regions below her eyes, a full face transplant may also include all the areas of the face—everything from the hairline down is replaced as if one were receiving a mask and not a simple skin graft. As extreme as such a procedure may sound, it is certainly within the bounds of surgical possibility, and indeed may have its benefits. Traditional graft procedures relocate portions of skin from another part of the body, often resulting in inconsistent skin texture that creates an array of apparitional problems, whereas transplanting the face of another person offers the transplant recipient actual facial skin tissue.

The advantage here, from medical and esthetic perspectives, is obvious. One might expect more face transplants since the advantages seem so great. However, matching a donor with a recipient is a difficult medical challenge. Of course, the surgeon must be prepared and skilled in the technique (face transplantations on cadavers have been practiced at both the Cleveland Clinic and the University of Louisville Kentucky).[3] However, there are additional physical issues related to blood match, gender, tissue compatibility, age of donor, and simply locating a donor. These are minimal requirements to satisfy the demands of ethics approval. The real crucial moment is when a donor match can move from the abstract to the concrete, allowing the procedure to occur. Even the removal of the donor face is a complicated procedure in which the donor must be brain dead, yet living on ventilation, to have the facial skin removed. Many pieces of a rather complicated puzzle must come together in order for a face transplant to occur. What coalesces is more or less a sort of perfect storm. For the recipient of the procedure, this perfect is only the start—a different storm will follow.

Even with the possibility of surgical perfection, there are complications of a nonsurgical, nonphysical nature that would threaten to undermine a successful face transplant. Yet, these issues have garnered little attention until recently. Over the past two years a great deal of academic research and scholarship has been centered on problems related to immunity or tissue rejection. Only recently have researchers and surgical teams begun to consider perhaps the most problematic aspect of face transplants, that is, the psychological. To lower the possibility of a person at psychological risk being administered a face transplant, face transplant teams are now focusing on psychological screening. Concerning a British transplant team, a recent *Observer* article noted, "one thing that the British team has learnt during the last two years is to concentrate on the psychological aspects as the key to selecting the right patients. The psychologist Alex Clarke has worked closely with Dr. Butler in both providing therapy for the patients and closely assessing their mental states."[4] This budding interest in psychological assessment does show a growing concern for the psychological import of face transplants. However, there is something else significant about the self that seems to escape even these psychological investigations into risk and acceptance assessment.

In the July 27, 2007, issue of *People* magazine, a one-page article updating the world on the status of Dinoire bore the headline, "It Will Never Be Me."[5] Many news articles written about Dinoire after her procedure have been rocked with reports of her unhappiness, depression, and struggles to adjust to her new appearance. However, this article in *People*, couched in praise for the new life her surgeons had given her, was the first time Dinoire hinted at the fact that she considered the procedure problematic. It will never be her? If her face was not her, or rather, her new face does not encapsulate what she was, then what is this "me" that Dinoire hints at? How does one begin to make sense of this apparitional aspect of her "self"? With all other questions that are raised by face transplant procedures, we can't help but feel that the question put to the self seems to trump all others.

Yes, face transplants are still relatively rare and remain far from being mainstream surgical procedures. Yet, the impending proliferation of face transplant procedures raises important cultural concerns at both practical and conceptual levels that so far have gone, for the most part, without comment. This void does contain the faint stirrings of commentary: questions of informed consent,[6] medical ethics,[7] and psychological appropriateness of clients, but, without a sustained theoretical attempt at construing the cultural significance of face transplants, the impact of the new procedure may remain obscure. This element of mystery could both jeopardize the future implementation of an innovative medical procedure, as well as possibly allow the procedure to continue to be performed without ethical direction. Such unabated movement would promise obvious dangers that the procedure might not obtain were the procedure given the proper consideration demanded by practical concern whenever society is pressed to adjust to a radical innovation. As the procedures continues to propagate, it is crucial to add a new set of questions to the chorus currently being mulled over concerning face transplant procedures.

An article on face transplantation on http://www.salon.com, in 1999, years before the first procedure took place, foreshadowed the concerns and questions raised after Dinoire: Will donors come forward? Will the procedure really work? Is it worth the risk of dosing a patient with immunosuppressive drugs to enhance appearance? Is it ethical to graft one human being's face onto the skull of another? Is it taboo?[8]

However, the article did not ask the more difficult questions: What does it mean for a face transplant to "work?" What is the relation of appearance to "self"? What does it mean to be ethical about face transplants? How does one even evaluate the ethics of a procedure that seems only to leave people shocked? If taboos have emerged in popular consciousness relating to face transplants, then how and why? Without answers to such questions, face transplants might irrevocably provoke grave psychological danger for their recipients by ignoring issues of disfigurement, the grotesque, and basic issues of human subjectivity.

Jean-Michel Dubernard, one of Isabelle Dinoire's surgeons, described the experience of looking at her before her surgery as "looking at life and death at the same time."[9] Dinoire still has a look that is hard to describe. There is something about trying to frame a face transplant that is rather like describing the experience of staring into the face of the sphinx; one just doesn't know what to say about it.

One way of beginning to interpret the procedure is to understand it as a story, which is to say, in terms of literature or mythology. As the myth and religion scholar Wendy Doniger has put it, "for many centuries, mythological texts have provided a kind of virtual reality testing ground for organ transplants: though it has become physically possible to do such operations only in recent decades, people have imagined, for a very long time indeed, the sorts of problems that might arise if one could do such things."[10]

As such a "testing ground," myths would provide a perfect place to start in understanding the unconscious attachments people seem to have to face transplants. The trouble is, there is not one simple myth concerned with face transplants, but a rich array of themes that can only be addressed through a number of different myths. Here in our introduction to this book, we briefly address three such myths.

An often overlooked myth of Ancient Greece, the myth of Marsyas, is the account of a musical contest that took place between Marsyas (a Phrygian satyr sometimes portrayed as a peasant) and the god Apollo. Marsyas is said to have come across a flute that was discarded by its inventor, the goddess Athena, after she was displeased with how playing the instrument affected her appearance. Having picked up Athena's flute, Marsyas came to compose much beautiful music. It is here that the myth tends to be taken up in two different manners, with two very different morals. In the first account, the contest is said to have occurred when Marsyas, suffused with overweening pride, challenged Apollo to the contest. In the other account, a much more humble Marsyas is said to have been challenged by Apollo after the god had become inflamed by jealous passion at the sound of Marsyas' music. In both accounts, however, Apollo bests Marsyas by demanding that the two figures attempt to play music upside down—not the best position for playing a woodwind instrument. What results in Marsyas' defeat is an element of the myth that both accounts agree on: Marsyas was then tied to a tree by Apollo and flayed alive, with the outpouring of his blood turned into the River Marsyas by pitying divinities.

Each tale seems to have a distinct moral: one related to human vanity, the other the feckless nature of the gods. Nonetheless, both stories share the idea that there is a certain limit to human achievement—be it in faith good or bad—beyond which no human should stray. Aside from the obvious link in the myth of Marsyas to face transplants—the theme of being flayed alive, the question of suffering fate as well as the vanity of humankind's accomplishments offers an excellent introduction to the idea of how face transplants allow human beings to exceed their place within their natural world. A face transplant challenges what people tend to take as the fundamental biological makeup of a person.

The story of Frankenstein, the monster with the brain and bodies of two different men brought back to life by science, is perhaps the best known modern myth that deals with the same question as the Marsyan myth. Whether it be Mary Shelley's early nineteenth-century novel, *Frankenstein: or, The Modern Prometheus* (in which Frankenstein was just "The Creature") or James Whale's controversial film adaptation for Universal in the early 1930s, the story of *Frankenstein* stands as one of the most profound cautionary tales regarding the dangers of science, technology, and the hubris of human beings. Built out of the tacit assumption that science is often deeply linked to a desire to control and dominate nature and reality, Shelley's tale, spun out in an impromptu fashion in front of guests of her very famous parents, addressed an anxiety of modernity that people still struggle with today. How much is humankind's fascination with technology a threat to its existence? In many ways, the Frankenstein myth serves as an inevitable backdrop for the staging of the world's first face transplant procedure. Regardless of the murkier issues that it stirs up, it is the tale of a doctor animating the dead through technology.[11] As such, it is a tale that stirs any reader to evaluate the benefits and drawbacks of new technology: what, for example, it means to truly be human and the feelings the shock of innovation provokes. Being a profound meditation on the nature of monstrosity, the Frankenstein myth even offers the opportunity (as is especially apparent in the early film version of Frankenstein starring Boris Karloff) to question what makes a monster: the nature of the beast or the fears that reside within us?

A more recent myth, perhaps fallen into obscurity, authored by a man still notorious for his discoveries and inventions, serves as the third myth in introducing the problems of face transplant procedures: Sigmund Freud's case study of Ida Bauer, who was better know to the world as "Dora." The case history of, arguably, the most important client of the founder of psychoanalysis, Dora is the tale of a woman whose life was wrought with the question who or what am I?[12] Dora traversed the impact of traumatic encounters. Her experiences included the disappointments connected to a father to whom she was deeply attached as well as the sexual advances from the husband of her father's mistress. Freud's analysis of Dora was an early attempt at substantiating many of his ideas about hysteria. His ideas included the exploration of her dreams, her somatic symptoms, and the powerful bonds of transference in analysis. Dora's problems persisted around an experience of instability in her sense of self-identity as a result of trauma. The relevance of such a tale for face transplant procedures lies in its description of the experience of doubting one's existence after a traumatic encounter. A doubt that functions less as a theological koan than it does as the experience of the loss of stability of what one's existence *means*. This trauma stands at the heart of the experience of receiving a face transplant. Although Freud was never quite able to resolve the identity problem for Dora, the case study nevertheless raised an interesting and ambiguous side of technology (if we can grant a technological status to the invention of psychoanalysis) that is not apparent in the work of Shelley: the trauma of the treatment itself. One should not forget that Freud's ideas had an effect he was aware of and anxious about, enough to have delayed the publication of his case study of Ida Bauer for several years.[13] If the treatment itself has an element of trauma to it, as the psychoanalytic understanding of reality certainly did and does for many patients, one must understand how this trauma can be both difficult and therapeutic at the same time.

Somewhere in the midst of these three myths there is something like the myth of a face transplant. Although, face transplant procedures have been performed in an incontestably successful manner, with three procedures having gone off more or less without a hitch, the complex feelings that the procedure has touched off (only hinted at by the Salon.com article cited above) border on the mythological. Beyond the initial shock that one feels at the idea of the procedure, one's imagination begins to run wild with associations and awe at the possibility of the procedure. Embedded in people's associations with face transplants, the various feelings of exuberance or fear that the procedure provokes offer ways of understanding what is difficult to swallow about the procedure. As Doniger points out, myth serves as the source material of our unconscious attitudes toward transplant procedures.[14]

Even though these three myths presented in this Introduction do not cleanly correspond to the chapters laid out in this book, their presence here affords us a look at three conversant themes serving as silent partners throughout this book: innovative technology, trauma, and identity. These three themes are certainly not the only issues that are present in the myths of Marsyas, Frankenstein, and Dora; however, no matter what other themes one finds in these stories, or even what other themes a person may associate with face transplants, the proper interpretation of a procedure as alluring and provocative as this one would go nowhere without their consideration.

Although the nature of trauma is a hotly contested issue in today's world, one aspect of trauma that transcends all debate is the way it is invariably experienced by individuals: as a disruption. The problem of trauma is the challenge of finding a way to make sense and incorporate an unprecedented experience in one's life—an experience that often includes an assortment of corporeal and psychological symptoms. In each myth evoked above, a character experiences a blunt intrusion into their world, forever changing it. The experiences leading a person to a face transplant are traumatic in nature (being the unfortunate recipient of some sort of disfiguring accident or intended violence). Despite the attempts of transplant teams who assess psychologically and choose the most healthy face transplant recipients, there is something about the experience of having the face of another person that may defy current assessment protocols. Throughout this book, we attempt to analyze the traumatic impact that the introduction of face transplant procedures seems to have had on people throughout the world, as well as on certain individuals who have been recipients of the procedure.

As much as this procedure and its response heralds an examination of the question of trauma, any trauma associated with the procedure would not have occurred without the advent of new and innovative technology. The myths discussed above each include the theme of innovation. They also speak to humankind's ability to create technology in one way or another (the flute, Frankenstein's lab, the psychoanalytic cure). An element of the trauma of face transplant procedures—both for an individual and for a culture—is obviously linked to the role technology has played in its application. As such, another major consideration of face transplant procedures is the role that innovative technology has played in their reception. The link between technology and trauma does not necessarily discount the good that technology might serve. Rather, by understanding trauma as having one's world disrupted, instead of pathology, the role of science is

expanded by encompassing both the pain of the disruption and its anodyne. Innovative transplant technologies can be understood as provoking
the bewildering admixture of emotions that people have emitted in
response to face transplants: fear and rejection, as well as overt enthusiasm.
Understanding how to interpret the new transplant technology could help
allay negative reactions to the procedure.

The third and most important theme addressed throughout this book,
indeed the focus and concern of our exploration, concerns the way trauma
and innovative technology challenge self-identity. The experience of something radically unprecedented raises grave questions about how we view
and understand the world around us. In each of the myths evoked above,
identity is challenged or affected through the experience of some trauma.
It may be the experience of losing something previously possessed or gaining something you did not want. The understanding of one's self is
impacted in all of the myths above, so too, it is challenged by face transplant procedures. We need to ask ourselves what it is about such surgery
that radically challenges how we look at ourselves as human beings and
challenges conventional ways of understanding identity.

The first chapter, "Unmasking the Face," reconstructs the history of
organ transplant procedures, in both their mythological origins, as well as
in their scientific accomplishments. By offering a chronology of organ
transplant procedures preceding face transplants, we ask questions about
the cultural development of transplant procedures throughout history. In a
sense, then, the history of transplant procedures (a story that one could
find elsewhere, for sure) is retold through the specific perspective of face
transplant procedures.

The second chapter, "Dreaming the Face," continues the mapmaking
spirit of the first chapter. Current cultural and social attitudes attached to
face transplant procedures are analyzed in relation to various cultural fantasies about them. The chapter begins with a small-scale qualitative exercise
that uncovers thematic anxieties about the procedures. The approach is
similar to a research methodology such as discourse analysis. The focus of
this relatively cutting-edge form of analysis is placed on finding more general contradictions, fears, and anxieties embedded in a collective storytelling exercise. Just as with our consideration of cultural anxieties and fears
expressed in popular culture, part of construing the limits of thought in a
collective narrative is to point to new ways of talking about face transplants
in academic discourse.

We follow our exploration of face transplant in cultural fantasies, with
two chapters that serve as a sustained attempt at using psychological and
psychoanalytic theory. Here we interpret the fantasy anxieties raised in the

previous chapter in light of questions of identity formation. As a mix of a person's "inner" and "outer" worlds, self-identity—the result of complicated developmental processes—is often explained in a drastically simplified manner. The function of these two chapters is dual: to elucidate aspects of certain psychoanalytic doctrines that are helpful in the interpretation of face transplant procedures, and to locate the limits of psychoanalytic reason in respect to the revelation of face transplant procedures. Without saying the final word on the topic, these chapters attempt to open up new ways of talking about identity that are, in some ways, novel to psychoanalytic theory itself.

The first of these two chapters, "Analyzing the Face: Part I," assumes the perspective of two developmental psychoanalytic approaches—the work of the British child psychoanalyst Donald Winnicott and of the French psychoanalyst Didier Anzieu—in talking about issues related to the human face and human skin. With special attention paid to the function of boundaries in identity formation, as well as their significance in face transplant procedures, this chapter offers a way of thinking about the anxiety of having one's identity interrupted, by looking at the psychosocial implications of one's skin as well as the role that faces play in the early life of children.

The second of this series of two chapters, "Analyzing the Face: Part II," continues the psychoanalytic exploration of the developmental formation of self-identity. Long one of the great perplexing and misunderstood concepts in psychoanalysis, Sigmund Freud's notion of symbolic castration serves as the cornerstone for his theory of development. This chapter examines the implications of the idea that a *cut* was what prompted identity formation and how this insight might be viewed in light of face transplant procedures. In so doing, this chapter also explores the interwoven nature of one's "outer" and "inner" worlds and the anchor point of a person's identity. While utilizing what is helpful in the Freudian understanding of identity formation, this chapter also takes the opportunity to point out what is problematic about it, ending by offering suggestions as to how one might refine and improve on the psychoanalytic understanding of identity as it arises in the case of face transplant procedures.

Picking up the theoretical discussion begun in the previous two chapters, the fifth chapter, "Narrating the Face," attempts to create a working theory of identity based on the premise that it is a complex narrative structure. Calling on a variety of understandings of narrative, stories, plot structure, and social movement drawn from philosophy and the social sciences, this chapter examines the ways in which the face interacts as a binding agent for the composite story that makes up the identity of individual human beings. This chapter casts the face in a variety of roles. It reconstructs the relationship between a face and an identity in a way that sheds light on the complications of face transplant procedures and how they might better function therapeutically in the life of a recipient. This chapter ends with encouraging words for the continuation of such procedures and offers insight into how surgeries might be performed more successfully by incorporating a more holistic approach. This approach might extend beyond surgery and into the process of the patient's attempt at adjusting to life with a new face.

Even with several face transplants having been completed since 2005 and with more looming on the horizon, the future use of face transplants is a question waiting to be answered. Electing to perform the procedure on a certain population of individuals—burn victims? animal attacks? genetic conditions?—will not only refine the specific ways that the procedure is performed (since certain conditions will demand different technical refinements), but will also define questions of policy and ethics. Because face transplant procedures are still experimental, their future is as yet undetermined.

The final chapter concludes our exploration. We ponder the possible use of face transplants on veterans of the armed forces who have been disfigured while serving in Iraq, Afghanistan, and elsewhere. As with every new war of the past two centuries, each war brings with it cutting-edge weaponry and technology that ends up creating new kinds of combat-related injuries for all of those involved. Although a long-standing adversary for veterans of war, disfigurement has risen to prominence during the current time of war, as it has been a major problem for many soldiers returning from the Middle East. Treatment of soldiers during this armed conflict has become somewhat of a hot-button issue in the popular press. A lot of pressure has fallen on medical communities to come up with ways of responding to contemporary war injuries and trauma. In addition to other technologically cutting-edge treatment methods, such as the use of virtual-reality therapy with war veterans suffering from posttraumatic stress disorder, face transplant procedures might serve a valuable purpose in aiding the effort to treat wounded and disfigured war veterans. As such, facial transplants could become a procedure specifically cultivated for use with disfigured soldiers.

This chapter also serves a secondary purpose: to revisit the three themes designated in the Introduction—trauma, innovative technology, and identity—in a contemporary context different from that of face transplants. Not only are these three issues pertinent to the experience of the wounded soldier, but the problem of war trauma as it relates to identity is a problem that will long outlast the duration of the current war in Iraq. Although our conjecture as to how face transplants may be taken up in the future could prove to be inaccurate, we have nevertheless considered the subject of this book's conclusion, Iraq War veterans and the problem trauma, as a fecund topic of consideration. Sharing both the thematic concerns of face transplant procedures as well as an uncertain future, a consideration of the intersection of face transplants and war-related injuries is a timely way to end this book's exploration, which is, in some sense, an exploration of what it means to be human at the beginning of the twenty-first century.

As hopeful face transplant surgeon Peter Butler told the British newspaper *Telegraph*, "Opinion is changing."[15] In the same spirit of change, we have one simple hope for this book: may it make you view the procedure, and the world itself, differently.

1

Unmasking the Face

Jacqueline Saburido is one of a number of individuals who have approached a face transplant team in England. She has an interest in receiving a partial transplant, after a car accident in Texas in 1999 left her severely disfigured. The car Jacqueline was traveling in was slammed into by an underage drunk driver and burst into flames. She was unable to escape, and more than 60 percent of her body was covered with third-degree burns. She was so severely injured that her fingers, lips, nose, and ears began to peel away from her body. In addition to the gruesome injuries that Jacqueline sustained in the accident were the additional scars of the medical procedures. Unknown to Jacqueline, the face with which she had grown up had been completely and irreparably lost.

Jacqueline lay in her hospital bed for months, enduring intense trauma-related symptoms, such as hallucinations that horses were trampling her and tearing away her skin. She did so without the full knowledge or extent of her injuries, which was only slowly revealed to her. She implored her supportive father to explain why she was no longer able to feel her fingers and consistently asked, "What do I look like? How is my hair? How is my skin?[1] Before the hospital psychological staff made plans to reveal the truth of her condition to her, Jacqueline began to catch on to the extent of her physical injuries when glimpsing a shadow given off by her transformed body. She had to deal with shock, yet persevered, displaying an improbably positive attitude. While she was participating in an extensive and ongoing treatment plan that included regular psychological counseling, reconstructive surgeries, the donning of a beige pressure suit, taking a costly daily array of medications, and having her skin salved with creams and medications to prevent skin tears and infections, she served as a spokesperson for a drunk-driving awareness campaign[2] and has even appeared as a guest on *The Oprah Winfrey Show*. Jacqueline was even eventually able to stand before the drunk driver who had so badly injured her. She admitted to the jury that she wanted to forgive him.

Saburido then began to take some of the most difficult steps in her complex journey of healing. The consequences of her injuries are still severe. Since 1999, she has undergone more than 50 procedures aimed at reconstructing the tissue on her face. Each process is arduous; the procedures have several times uprooted her from where she lives. She is still only about halfway complete, and she has persisted in pursuing differing avenues of treatment. She has approached the British face transplant team, led by reconstructive surgeon Peter Butler; she has also appeared in several documentaries, not merely to raise awareness about her story, but also as an advocate and an active seeker of a face transplant.

Jacqueline's wish raises the interesting question—should a face transplant be preferred to standard reconstructive surgery, the process she has already started? The question whether it is worth performing a single major procedure that might "reconstruct" Jacqueline's face, as opposed to a long series of reconstructive surgeries, does not have an immediate and clear answer. These are technically difficult and dangerous procedures. Despite what is initially jarring about allotransplantations—wearing a body piece of another, face transplants offer many benefits. In spite of the risks of tissue rejection that would be involved with a face transplant, there are benefits, especially from experiencing only a small number of procedures as opposed to the nearly one hundred that are necessitated by the reconstruction process. A face transplantation functions and appears to be a human face. No matter how well crafted the traditional skin graft is performed, the usual reconstruction process is arguably less convincing and less serviceable in the role of the face.[3]

Reconstruction may be debated along more or less technical lines, but when confronted with an individual such as Jacqueline Saburido, a young woman deprived of her normal appearance, any real debate would feel contrived. She is the most compelling of cases for a face transplant, as well as an ideal recipient for the procedure. Her attitude remains remarkably positive, in an interview or reading her posts from her Web site; her plea for a face transplant seems transparent and convincing, and yet, perhaps not compelling enough for other people. Even when presented with as an extraordinary an individual as Jacqueline is, someone so positive, someone who has persevered through incredible adversity, there are still many people skeptical as to whether face transplants should be performed. When confronted with such an obvious matter, what would motivate such skepticism? Doubts over the implementation of face transplant procedures very rarely stem from technical, medical, or professional–ethical perspectives, and more typically stem from elsewhere, such as religious beliefs or culture.[4] Such views prevent people from endorsing a procedure, even for obvious recipients.

It would seem that the vast majority of fears and doubts related to transplant procedures stem from general misinformation over the topic; the source of this—be it neglect or belief—is less clear.

Attempts to navigate the fears associated with the medical-technological change that comes with a face transplant demand that such neglect of information be corrected. Part of this correction must first be arrived at through a historical reading of the emergence of face transplant procedures that does not imply the facts involved with its past, but also an inquiry pertaining to the ideas that have fostered the historical development of transplant procedures; this does not simply state the facts but also is an inquiry into the ideas that have fostered the development of transplant procedures. These notions have been well described in fields such as sociology, anthropology, and cultural studies,[5] but a history of transplant procedures gleaned through the prism of face transplants leaves one with a markedly different outlook when contrasted with other histories. To understand face transplant procedures, where they now stand and where they are perhaps headed, we must first establish where face transplants have come from. That is, one must understand the legacy of face transplants as a transplant procedure within medicine and culture. Indeed, within the history of transplant procedures leading up to the first face transplants at the start of the twenty-first century, there seems to be a story of growth, a story that has concerned both humankind's ability to challenge and overcome certain scientific problems of the body, as well as more fundamental questions concerning the nature of the self implied by existing in the unique form that human beings do. After the first U.S. face transplant, lead surgeon Maria Siemionow commented to the media that "to face the world, you need a face." Without face transplant procedures, however, this story of the face and identity cannot be told. The moment that faces could be swapped surgically, an entirely new story of the human body and of identity began to emerge.

RECONSTRUCTION

Each year in the United States an estimated seven million people require composite tissue reconstruction.[6] Surgical excision of tumors, accidents, and congenital malformations often leave large and unwieldy wounds requiring the repair of many types of anatomical structures. Nerves, blood vessels, muscles, bone, and skin, different composites, must undergo repair. Historically, reconstructive surgeons had the daunting task of mending these surgically created wounds using the patient's own body. Some of the most medically complex repairs are performed on severe burns to the body or face. Burn injuries to the face, in particular, can be some of the most heartbreakingly challenging for both patient and doctor. Consider the psychological fate of facial burn patients. First, they suffer the stress and horror of the wound. Then, their sense of identity is grossly disrupted. Even loved ones and acquaintances must relearn the new face. Medically, facial burn patients must cope with pain and the time involved with replacing their body or facial skin. Typically, skin is taken from locations with large available areas, such as the thigh and back. Reconstructive surgeons describe burn repair procedures as "life by 1,000 cuts." It is not uncommon for a treatment to involve up to 80 or 90 reparative operations. Cuts must be made at both the harvest and transplant locations. The results are unfortunately never entirely esthetically pleasing. Skin from one's back or thighs simply never acts or looks like facial skin. The procedure oddly leaves every facial burn patient with an identical uniform, patch-worked, quilted, and tight-skinned look. Often in the case of a severe facial burn, as there was with Saburido, there is the complete loss of facial details, such as ears, lips, and nose. Unfortunately, even the most talented reconstructive surgeons of today have not mastered perfecting duplicates of these deceptively simple human features.

When a reconstruction is attempted, say of the ear, some of the patient's own body can only supply the most basic materials. Cartilage, for example, can be harvested and used for reconstruction, leaving two wound sites to heal. In some cases, big toes have been transplanted onto hands to serve as thumbs. That kind of procedure is quite rare and necessitates completely sacrificing one piece of the body in an exchange for another, not an ideal solution by any means.[7] In the case of facial burn patients, the best solution and ultimate fantasy is to replace "like with like"—the reconstructive surgeon's mantra. In an interview with the English newspaper *Guardian* British plastic surgeon Peter Butler commented on the first time he fantasized about the possibility of a face transplantation. He was only twenty-four years old and had just encountered a young burn patient:

> His lips were hanging down, he was dribbling, he had lost his nose and his ears, the skin around the eyes was stretched down so he couldn't look forward. "It was hard for him to leave the house because the injuries were so bad that people couldn't bear to look at him. And I just thought that there had to be something better for a boy like him. I felt that as doctors we had to work to try and give him some kind of future.[8]

Today Butler is originator and director of The Face Trust. This London-based charity helps to raise public awareness about face transplantation. It also works to solicit funds to support the expensive transplant procedure. Currently Butler is one of a handful of reconstructive surgeons worldwide who are approved to perform facial transplantations.

LEGEND OF THE BLACK LEG

Amazingly, it was in approximately 300 AD that the first recorded composite tissue allotransplantation occurred.[9] A composite tissue transplantation (CTA) is defined as any mismatched genetic material taken from one person's body and attached to someone else that involves a composite or combination of tissues, such as bone, nerves, blood vessels, skin, muscles, and so on. As the legend goes, twin brothers from Arabia, Saints Cosmas and Damian, amputated the gangrenous leg of a suffering temple guard and replaced it with a limb from the corpse of an Ethiopian man. This extraordinarily early attempt to allotransplant a suffering man's limb with a dead man's limb was truly a moving tribute aimed at alleviating brutal suffering through technological compassion. Saints Cosmas and Damien must have known that the procedure was ultimately destined for failure, yet their achievement was indeed prescient. Across the history of medicine one can only imagine how alluring the fantasy must have been of just taking one needed piece off another person and replacing it with a like part from another. Replete with bone, nerves, arteries, and skin, this kind of transplantation would not inflict pain nor endanger the donor in anyway whatsoever and would spare the recipient the risks associated with harvesting parts from their own body. Clearly there is a significant degree of pain and suffering avoided with an allotransplantation.

To give one an idea of how entirely premature this operation was, it would not be until approximately 1,600 years later that one man's hand was successfully transplanted onto another. In 1998, the first successful composite tissue allograft procedure was performed in France. To bring even more perspective, as of 2008, leg allotransplantations have yet to be successfully performed on a human, there have only been a couple dozen human hand transplantations (many of those were double hand transplants), and only four successful human facial allografts have been performed.[10]

HISTORICAL RECONSTRUCTION

The history of transplantation procedures can be unfolded in a number of ways. There can be a straight recounting of the events as they occurred year by year or some kind of conceptual and organizing framework can be imposed on the telling of a historical story. Here, the story of transplantations accomplishes both a straight recounting of transplants across history and offers a conceptual framework that provides a deeper understanding. One way to organize the historical material into a subtext is to demonstrate that the kinds of transplants themselves have emerged in a pattern that echoes other cultural movements underway, such as art, philosophy, music, science, and literature. While it is outside our purpose here to explore all of culture, it is argued that transplant procedures follow an outside/inside/outside pattern. In other words, the very earliest transplants involved concerns about the outside surfaces of bodies, for example, missing noses and as we have already mentioned limbs. Historically, the next advancements in transplant procedures moved from the outside surface of the body to the inside of the body where harvesting and the transplantation of solid tissue organs progressed. More recently, the cutting edge of contemporary transplant allotransplantations is with smaller internal body parts such as trachea, peripheral nerve, knees, larynx, abdominal wall, and even a tongue,[11, 12] and has advanced, once again, to the exteriors of bodies most notably with face transplantations.

SKIMMING THE SURFACE

Early history of transplantations involved Gaspare Tagliacozzi (1547–1599), considered by many to be the father of modern plastic surgery, who transferred a nose from a slave to his master.[13, 14] The early procedures involved the repair of noses missing because of trauma or syphilis. Even as early as the sixteenth century, skin was routinely scraped off the face to rebuild the nose. Others developed techniques where the upper arm skin could be utilized in replacing the nose. Many of these procedures required that patients keep their forearms bandaged to their faces until the skin healed and adhered. Other early uses of facial reconstruction included correcting ethnic-looking eyes and noses or simply restoring the human form back to pre-injury state.

The modern day focus on the outside of the body began around World War I when about a half a million men were treated for facial injuries sustained in the trenches. Soon after, incredible advances emerged in the surgical world, in particular the administration of anesthesia, instrument sterilization, hand washing, and simply the tremendous growth in surgical techniques developed while helping millions of troops afflicted by the ravages of a war fought in the trenches. War has always been good for the learning and advancing of surgical techniques. In this war the injuries were particularly daunting. Dealing with combat wounds inflicted by potent ammunition on soldiers in stationary situations like trenches permitted surgeons to try novel and more effective surgical methods. Also, deeper wounds meant more experience with the insides of bodies, and this permitted the development of techniques that would permit transplantations taken from the inside of bodies.

DEEPER INTO ORGANS

After a shift change from looking and surveying and lightly digging under the surface to digging deeper into organs, perhaps the most famous of transplants, by Joseph Murray, occurred in Boston in 1954.[15] Murray, a plastic surgeon, performed the first human kidney transplant between identical twin brothers on December 23 of that year. The twins were identical; therefore threats of rejection were greatly diminished. There was no genetic mismatch with which to contend, and no antirejection drugs were necessary. The transplant caused a remarkable storm of media attention and criticism. In the popular media, Murray was accused of playing God and of tampering with nature, but those in the medical field were greatly encouraged, and in many ways it was Murray's kidney transplantation that signaled a turning point and a kind of cultural end bud. What for so long had just been a fantasy now became a reality—like with like! Once Murray sutured the transplant wound closed on that December day, he sealed up an important cultural dynamic along with it—the age of diving beneath the surface begins to close and the challenges of surfaces again reawakens. Of course following the first successful kidney transplant in 1954, there were many other firsts: heart (1967), liver (1967), lung (1983), and heart/lung (1986). The success of the internal solid organ allotransplantations was completely dependent on the development of the immunosuppressant drug cyclosporine. Developed in a laboratory in Switzerland during the 1970s, it was discovered that this soil-borne fugal bacteria worked to reduce the body's immunologic response to allotransplanted tissues. In the 1990s, the drug tacrolimus was developed in Japan and approved for use in transplantations. Both of these drugs decreased the risk of death from allotransplantations so dramatically that their use has practically begun to seem routine to the public. Both medications carry a very long list of side effects that must be endured for the life of the patient. Specifically the various and common side effects range from the manageable but debilitating such as headaches, hypertension, diarrhea, and vomiting to very serious but more infrequent problems like cancer. Without the medications however organ rejection is inevitable and recipients face another transplant or death.

Great advances in pharmacology and surgical technology have permitted some innovative reconstructive surgeons to return to the preoccupation of Saints Cosmas and Damien. Composite tissue allotransplantation reignites dreams of joining surfaces of bodies, bringing to the surface complex questions such as racial identity and the meanings inherent in body interchangeability.

RESURFACING

It is significant that the patron saints of surgeons in the Roman Catholic tradition are in fact the Saints Cosmas and Damien. Transplants are in some ways the single most important kind of surgery because they speak to not only very deep levels of compassion, but also how they open up thought and discussion about psychological dimensions of inside and outside rejection, boundaries, and identity. It is here that the story turns to two kinds of allotransplantation firsts, specifically of the hand and face. These grafts, perhaps more than any other, take on related issues of boundaries, fears of rejection, and identity by forcing on us a kind of difficult psychologically based discussion vis-à-vis the real problems inherent in such operative procedures. Consider the idea of donor match for skin type. Not only must the donor match the recipient for blood type and antigens as is necessary for internal solid organs, but now, more esthetic issues such as skin color, density, texture, gender, age, and race must be seriously considered. Consider the problems of a man's hand or face on a woman's body, and it becomes apparent why many still consider face transplantation a cosmetic procedure. If facial allografts, for example, were completely for life-saving functions, these kinds of "look" matters would be less pressing. Face transplantation takes issues related to gender, race, and age to a new level and heightens awareness of how complex identity truly is. Harvard Medical School professor Bohdan Pomahac has been told from potential face transplant patients he has interviewed that they are so desperate to receive a normal-looking face that they would accept a face of another color.[16] Certainly this makes one wonder not only about racial identity and the meaning of the face, but also about even more complex issues about the nature of identity—the flexibility of identity in particular.

THE FIRSTS

The first hand transplantation was attempted in Ecuador in February 1964.[17] Unfortunately, two weeks after the procedure the hand showed the first signs of rejection and had to be amputated. In many ways the attempt was premature. Technically speaking microsurgery was still under development, and it was not until 1976 that cyclosporine A was introduced and ushered in a new era of transplantation.[18] Cyclosporine-based immunosuppression regimens caused acute rejection rates in transplants to fall from above 70 percent to less than 50 percent.[19] In the late 1970s and early 1980s three groups tested the efficacy of cyclosporine A in upper extremity transplants in primates. Although rejection was suppressed for periods of up to 300 days in these experiments, the highly immunologic skin portions of transplanted extremities were rejected within the first few months and had to be removed.[20, 21, 22] It is important to realize that much of what would later plague, and to some extent still haunts, face transplant surgeons were these early research reports rigorously stating that skin somehow seemed to be a different entity when it came to allotransplantation. If the skin was indeed more susceptible to rejection, then hand and face allotransplantations would be a much more difficult sell to reconstructive surgeons. After all, the burden of convincing formidable hospital institutional review boards would be compounded if surgeons could not reassure them that there was enough reassuring research stating that working with allotransplanted skin would not cause unique problems. Until these skin-related immunological issues could be addressed more convincingly through research or otherwise, any allotransplantation involving the use of skin would have to wait. Thus, between discouraging laboratory results with limb allotransplantations and the failed human hand allograft in Ecuador, reconstructive surgeons abandoned further attempts to transplant a human hand for almost another three decades.

JUST DO IT

In 1991, a conference was held to discuss the clinical use of CTA. The meeting was held in conjunction with the Rehabilitation Research and Development Service of the Department of Veterans Affairs in Washington, D.C., specifically to see if it was feasible to transplant limbs in patients. Questions such as if limbs could be transplanted from one patient to another were discussed. The group concluded with great optimism and even predicted that by 1995 there would be tremendous practical advances seen in the field.[23] However, six years later in November 1997 when the First International Symposium on CTA was held in Louisville, Kentucky, no significant practical changes in the field had occurred. At the meeting a discussion was held speaking of "the barriers standing in the way of performing human hand transplants." The talks primarily focused on immunologic and ethical barriers to performing hand transplantations. Near the end of the conference it was declared by John Barker, the lead surgeon on the allotransplantation team at Louisville, and others that enough animal research had been done and it was time to "just do it."[24] This positive "just do it" shout from middle America may very well have been responsible for pushing forward the innovative surgeries that were to occur within the next ten years, beginning with the first successful hand allograft.

Despite the enthusiasm of the Louisville team, they were not the first to perform the procedure. Instead, a team that was unknown to Barker and his Kentucky colleagues suddenly announced in September 1998 that they had performed the first hand allotransplantation in France. Barker was later quoted as being very surprised to learn of the French-based team because he had never heard of the group and they had not participated in the discussions from the year before. The Louisville team however did perform the first U.S. hand transplantation in January 1999. These two hand allotransplantations were historic and successful at both the level of surgical skill and at immunosuppressant levels. Furthermore, because the transplants involved a large degree of donated skin, this encouraged doctors to become more confident in the potential for facial allotransplantation. Barker made the following comment concerning the relationship between hand and face transplantations: "Perhaps the single most important development that allowed facial transplantation to be considered as clinically feasible was the early success of human hand transplantation. Many of the same technical, immunologic, psychosocial and ethical barriers that were overcome to perform human hand transplants served to pave the way for performing human facial transplants."[25] The story of the first successful hand allotransplantation is intriguing and in fact, full of intrigue at many levels.

FIRST SUCCESSFUL HAND ALLOTRANSPLANTATION

Surgical teams in France, the United States, and Australia were arguably tacitly vying to perform the first hand allotransplantation. The winning team, so to speak, would require a kind of perfect storm to occur with the following three vital elements: 1) a large degree of professional bravado; 2) a patient willing and capable of weathering the inevitable related health risks, heavy media scrutiny, and loss of privacy; and 3) the creation of an ethical informed consent form.

The Surgeon

The professional bravado component would materialize in the form of redoubtable French reconstructive surgeon Jean-Michel Dubernard. Dubernard was certainly no stranger to the public, having served as a Deputy in the French Parliament since 1986. In addition he worked as a physician for patients at the Edouard Herriot Hospital in Lyon, the very hospital in which he was born. His medical training began at the University of Lyon and then continued on to a research position in Belgium where he conducted research on liver and other transplants. While in Belgium, Dubernard was interested in a temporary research trainee position at Harvard University with Joseph E. Murray of kidney transplant fame. Ultimately he was accepted by the Boston team at the age of twenty-four when no one else would take the position. Dubernard's medical training concluded in Lyon where he did his doctoral work on xenotransplantations, that is, transplants between two different species such as kinds of monkeys. At the age of thirty-seven he became chief of urology at the Herriot Hospital and at the University of Lyon.[26]

The media's depiction of Dubernard usually highlights aspects of his strong personality, especially his bravado. He has been said to "love the limelight,"[27] and as rushing into the transplant for fame and celebrity,[28] and "seeking notoriety on media talk shows and the press."[29] Ultimately, even those somewhat critical of Dubernard's "rush" to perform the first hand transplant understood that the bravado component of his personality was necessary to get the first transplant underway. Peter Butler of London's Royal Free Hospital was planning to perform the world's first, not partial but full face transplantation. When he heard that Dubernard had performed the first face transplantation many years after the hand, he commented that although he would not have operated on Isabelle Dinoire, he still "applaud[ed] them in the sense that at some point someone had to move ahead and just do it."[30] With his go-for-it attitude, Dubernard sought suitable hand transplant candidates from outside of France, leading him into collaboration with surgeon Earl Owen of Australia and Owen's patient, Clint Hallam. Together Dubernard and Owen assembled the international surgical team to replace the New Zealander's missing forearm and hand.

The Patient

The first successful hand transplant recipient was forty-eight-year-old New Zealander Clint Hallam. Hallam's home surgeon Australian Earl Owen reported that while his team was well prepared to perform the first hand transplantation on his home territory, his team was having trouble finding a donor—in part due to negative public sentiment and the sheer scarcity of locating a donor of the forearm and hand. Owen hoped that France's population at 58 million compared to Australia's population of 18.6 million, along with its generous organ donor program would increase the odds of locating a donor match. In France one is assumed to be an organ donor unless otherwise stated. Although Dubernard was flush with potential donors, he was short of those requiring and requesting to be a hand allo-graft recipient. Thus, for practical concerns more than anything else, Owen and Hallam traveled with high hopes of having the procedure performed in France.

Attendant with the first hand transplantation, and helpful in under-standing the controversies surrounding issues related to being first, were many accusations that Hallam had been misrepresented to the French sur-gical team, perhaps as a way to make him seem as desirable and deserving as possible. The French team was told that Hallam was "a New Zealand businessman aged 48 years who had moved to Australia and who had had a traumatic circular-saw amputation of his right forearm in 1984."[31] However, it was later revealed that Hallam was actually not only in prison at the time of his circular saw mishap but was also wanted in a Western Australian court for seven counts of fraud and that he had led a life of petty crime. Dubernard later conceded that although he felt his team had been misled as to the character of his patient, that "as a doctor, I take care of everybody and did not change anything," stating that Hallam "desperately wanted the graft."[32] Oddly, even Hallam's own home surgeon Owen confessed that he had been "duped for two years" and added that Hallam "is a consummate rogue."[33] Nevertheless the operation was per-formed at the Edouard Herriot Hospital in Lyon, France, by an interna-tional surgical team of hand, orthopedic, and transplant surgeons, all skilled in microsurgical techniques and assembled specifically for Hallam's allograft.[34]

As part of his preparation for the operation Hallam underwent a battery of mental health assessment tests by both a French psychiatrist and psycho-analyst. In addition, the surgical team requested that Hallam conduct cer-tain exercises that would prepare his forearm muscles for the operation. For example, when it was discovered that Hallam had once played the piano, the medical experts suggested that he should pretend to play the musical instrument to help prepare the forearm for the transplantation. Hallam reported many phantom-limb syndrome events such as pain and sensations in the missing limb that were interpreted as positive signs that there were still active neural pathways between his arm and his brain. This boded well for postoperative functioning.[35] The surgical team assembled, examined Hallam, and waited with hopes the donor would fortuitously materialize. Unfortunately, a donor did not appear during this period of preparation, and the transplant team began to slowly disperse to attend to other business. A few days after they had split up a notice arrived that they should make their way back to Lyon for the surgery, an appropriate donor of the forearm and hand had arrived at the hospital.

Consent

The consent form was possibly the biggest stumbling block in many ways. The risk here was not medical in nature per se, but the ethical problem of creating an informed consent document that would permit the best possible information about the risks associated with the first hand transplantation—obviously a challenging task.[36] For example, agreeing to a life-long regiment of toxic, even potentially cancer-causing imunnosuppressant drugs is routine for kidney or heart transplantation recipients. But, a hand transplantation is considered more of a life-enhancing, rather than life-saving, operation. An ethics form would have to explain that the risks of drug-related complications were high for a procedure that might be greatly desired, but not life saving. An additional concern requiring introduction in the consent form was the possibility that the hand, like any transplanted organ, could undergo irreversible physical rejection. Complicating matters were that the odds of rejection were completely unknown because hand allotransplantation in the age of cyclosporine was untried. The patient, in addition, had to be informed of the very real and possibly stressful effects of intense media scrutiny after the operation. Related were the possible myriad of psychological repercussions associated with the long-term wearing of the hand of another—this was something nobody really knew anything about.

The right cocktail had been concocted. There was an outspoken excellent surgeon co-leading the team, a formidable patient who, with his criminal past, was presumably tough enough to weather whatever storm was ahead for him, and a good enough consent form.

Hand Transplantation

Hallam's donor was a brain-dead forty-one-year-old man who had suffered a traumatic head injury. He was a good match for Hallam's blood type, antigens, age, and skin. Hallam was notified and quickly prepared for the surgery. Details of the transplant procedure were reported in the medical journal *The Lancet*. The transplant process commenced with the removal of the donor's forearm and hand from just above the elbow. The appendage was then irrigated with an organ preservation solution. The donor's missing arm was replaced with a "custom-made aesthetic prosthesis, which was provided to restore normal appearance."[37] In this way, the world's first successful hand transplantation donor was laid to rest.

Hallam's forearm stump was then painstakingly prepared to receive the donated arm. The success of the microsurgery procedure would depend on how well the available muscles and neurovascular structures could be dissected, identified, and tagged.[38] The transplant surgery itself began with the screwing together of the two bones in the forearm: the donor's ulna and radius to the recipient. Arteries and veins were then sutured together, followed by the release of a clamp holding back the blood supply. Although twelve hours had elapsed between the time of the donor's death and when the tourniquet was released, "the hand rapidly achieved normal colour."[39] Next, the nerves were microsutured together and the donor's muscles and tendons were attached to Hallam's. It was discovered during this phase of the surgical process however that the donor's thumb was most likely impossible to repair because of some "hypothetical possible degree of preexisting thumb malfunction."[40] There really is no way to know what this information must have meant to the attending surgeons. It can only be surmised that the information must have been a disappointment. After all, this precious donated gift was perhaps not going to be able to be as functional as presumed. Ultimately "a decision was made not to divert other muscles to activate the thumb because of the pre-existing slight first-web-space contracture on the donor hand."[41] In other words, inside the webbed space between the thumb and first finger existed damage to the extent that it would most likely leave Hallam without an effective opposable thumb.

In the final steps of the operation, Hallam's skin was sutured together with the donor's skin, and then the arm and wrist were set in a splint to heal. The hand itself was left exposed for observation. Postsurgical treatment consisted of the introduction of the typical antibiotics and blood thinners given to most surgery patients. Hallam was also begun on a course of the immunosuppressant drug tacrolimus and steroids to prevent rejection. Physiotherapy was begun ten hours after surgery and then continued twice daily for the entire follow-up period. Action and motion exercises were performed as well as an "early sensory reeducation and cortical regeneration protocol."[42] The world's first successful hand allotransplantation was thus complete.

Physical Rejection

It is not uncommon for transplant patients to experience mild to moderate signs of rejection. Around eight weeks after the surgery Hallam's antirejection drugs were reduced, and he soon experienced a bout of redness in the graft that necessitated an increase of his tacrolimus. Up to this point, it had been assumed by transplant surgeons that skin possessed a higher immunosuppressant response than other parts of the human body. Nevertheless, the hand graft actually proved to be easier to manage because of the simple fact that signs of rejection could be quickly spotted and treated. Soft organ body transplants may begin signs of rejection that are detected too late, whereas skin rejections can be immediately treated, avoiding more harrowing consequences. In this case, a topical immunosuppressant ointment was initiated. Within three days, the combination of immunosuppressant drug and topical ointment completely eliminated all signs of rejection.

Psychological Rejection

Three years after the operation Hallam became uncomfortable with the transplanted hand and failed to follow the postoperative drug and physiotherapy program aimed at maintaining the transplant. His body slowly started rejecting the hand. The transplanted allograft was removed at his request on February 2, 2001, by one of the surgeons on his original transplant team. Hallam's refusal to keep the hand received very limited attention in the medical literature. When it was mentioned, it was usually attributed to some general term such as medical "noncompliance." The majority of literature concerning hand allotransplantation, following Hallam' transplant, is very upbeat in tone. For example, the team from the International Registry of Hand and Composite Tissue Transplantation reported that between 1998 and 2006 eighteen patients underwent twenty-four hand/forearm/digit transplantations and that all patients were men. The report noted a 100 percent patient survival rate, stating that the grafts did well, and all instances of problems, such as mild signs of rejection and infection, were successfully treated. However, for the majority of hand transplant patients, functional results have been quite impressive. "All viable hands presented normal skin color and texture, as well as normal hair growth and nail growth ... [and] all patients [could] perform grasp and pinch activities."[43] Most of these patients had returned to work and in 83 percent of the cases attested that they felt that the quality of life had been improved.[44] The most negative report from China reported that seven Chinese hand allograft patients did not have access to their immunosuppressant drugs and their grafts thereafter failed and had to be amputated.

Clint Hallam's request to have the first successfully completed allograft removed marked the transition from medical, immunological, and surgical technique concerns dominating the literature to more ethical and psychological concerns. If, for example, the surgical techniques and regime of medications were no longer the hurdles, the medical world had to somehow reconcile Hallam's psychological rejection of the transplanted hand. There were two explanations for why he rejected the hand: one, that he was a bad patient (note bad person can easily be woven into this perspective considering his checkered past), for example, he would not take his medicines out his "rogueness"; and two, that he had preexisting undetected psychological issues that contributed to his rejection of the donated hand. Notably missing here are any fruitful discussions that having the hand of another would be just unacceptable, creepy, or simply unwanted. A BBC news report from 2000 reported that Hallam was "distressed by how many people, even close friends, avoid him because they find his new hand repulsive."[45] If one chooses, for example, not to take the immunosuppressant drugs, then every patient very well knows that the hand will begin to be rejected. Interestingly, in an article published immediately after Hallam's allograft, he is discussed in the most robust sounding of mental health terms. Such as, "the patient refused available aesthetic or functional prostheses and preferred to read relevant studies and make himself available to [hand transplant] units contemplating limb transplantation."[46] In addition, the surgeons who authored the initial medical report remarked that there were certainly risks to taking a lifetime of immunosuppressant drugs for a "functional non-vital part of the body." In response to the risk, they continued, "our recipient took the initial decision autonomously, while in good mental health and able to balance an improvement in the quality of life against the potential risk of morbidity and mortality."[47] In fact, John Barker at Louisville admitted that Hallam had been on his request list.[48] Although not an indication of mental health per se, it does speak to Hallam's level of motivation and of his competence to locate surgical teams worldwide that were prepared to perform hand transplantations. It bears repeating that the donated hand had a defective thumb, and it can be speculated that the hand itself simply may not have functioned in a satisfactory manner, inducing a poor psychological outlook.

THE PENIS TRANSPLANT

The first and thus far only successful penis allotransplant procedure was performed on September 2006 at a military hospital in Guangzhou, China. The forty-four-year-old patient had sustained the loss of his penis in a traumatic amputation. The transplanted penis came from a brain-dead twenty-two-year-old. Although the operation was considered successful and he could urinate normally after the surgery, the patient and his wife were not satisfied with the results. Both the recipient and wife requested that the organ be removed, simply citing that although it functioned well enough, that they did not like it.[49] Considering that the transplant in this case was a penis, few really questioned why wearing the penis of another would be psychologically difficult. Unlike in Hallam's case, few accusations were launched of the recipient's or recipient's wife's psychological status.

One medical article did mention, upon reflection of the penis transplant rejection, that there was once again a "need for careful psychological screening in recipients and families in composite tissue allografts."[50] Again, one needs to consider that a negative response to any donated organ may be understood in a couple of ways. That is, rejection could be interpreted as a sign of bad citizenship (a bad person) or of poor psychological health. Ultimately, it may all depend on what kind of external organ is received. This will be an interesting area of allotransplantation to watch unfold as more transplants are performed. However, clearly, Hallam's case was the first to trigger grave concerns related to the wearing of another's body part. His case should be viewed as helpful, as a red flag warning that indeed allotransplantations could be psychologically disturbing.

Less then ten years after Hallam gained and removed his donated hand, Isabelle Dinoire would receive her facial allotransplantation. No one knew, not her surgeons, not herself, and not psychologists how she might relate to wearing the face of another. In many ways, to understand the meaning of a new face, it is necessary to understand the significance of the face itself.

FACING UNDERSTANDING

It has been argued that facial allografts are cosmetic and not life saving. That is, that face transplants serve the purpose of beautifying the face, more than saving the life of the recipient. However, faces carry with them very deep seated meanings that cross the medical, into the psychological and social realms of each human. Michael Eigen, a New York–based psychoanalyst and prolific author, features a chapter on the face in his book *The Electrified Tightrope*. The section called "The Significance of the Face" begins with this sentence: "The centrality of the human face as symbolic of personality permeates the fabric of human experience."[51] He speaks, for instance, of the infant's gaze into the mother's face while nursing. Here, he suggests, a permanent link is forged between faces and pleasure.

In 1990 Macgregor published a classic study outlining the major social problems that people with facial disfigurements endured.[52] The study is really quite telling, suggesting that facially disfigured folks habitually experienced harrowing problems such as social distancing, shunning, and teasing. In the year 2004, one year before the first face transplant, the *International Journal of Surgery* published a series of commentaries presenting a variety of social and psychological considerations pertaining to face transplantation.[53] Farrer, for example, suggested that a transplanted face might trigger a negative social response tantamount to those with a facial deformity. Because one never gets full neurological functioning in a facial allograft, the transplanted face may be experienced as socially unresponsive. Thus, "the outcome might not be physical rejection per se but could well leave the patient socially rejected as odd, inexpressive or 'cold.'"[54] In fact, the present technique for helping facial burn victims usually involves replacing the skin with flaps taken from other areas of the body such as the arm, buttocks, back, or thighs and then placing them patchwork-like onto the face. This technique, while providing the face with skin that performs basic epidermal functions, can never be esthetically pleasing. Simply put, the process creates a face that is inexpressive and immobile. Dinoire commented that she wanted a new face precisely so that she could show emotions. The two emotions she craved, but was denied by her excessive injury, were grimacing and smiling. Although not many conclusions can be drawn by the comment alone, it is compelling to think why those affects seemed most relevant and missed. It may be surmised that expressing to others what one enjoys or wishes to avoid may be elemental to our make-up—the deepest psychic cut in many ways: expressing one's likes and dislikes. Our ability to share with others the joy we feel when being with them or to express our dislikes are the basic building blocks of social intimacy. It is also possible that simply by not being able to move one's facial muscles into a smile or grimace prevents one from experiencing those emotions beyond the faintest of sparks. If the facial feedback hypothesis is correct, this would exactly be the case.

Facial feedback theory suggests that we cannot feel emotion without the benefit of receiving certain neurological signals from our facial muscles. In other words it is not the emotion of feeling happy that makes one smile, but rather the muscular formation of a grin that sends messages to the brain that causes feelings of happiness. Likewise, if you make a face, such as a frown, it has been demonstrated that this facial configuration will cause you to feel sad.[55] There is one very rare medical condition called Mobius syndrome where infants are born without the ability to make facial expressions. This disorder is a helpful test of the facial feedback hypothesis. After all, folks with Mobius cannot smile, frown, or move most of their face in any way—a lot like a facial burn patient who has been repaired with a patchwork of unyielding skin.

Jonathan Cole's book *About Face* is one of the only books to deal extensively with the social aspects of Mobius syndrome. In it he interviews those who live with the affliction and describes how they have experienced the social world around them. The disorder itself is named after the German neurologist Paul Mobius (1853–1907). The syndrome is marked by the presence of normal facial muscles but with a dysfunction of the nerves to move the muscles. Individuals who have the disorder suffer from different degrees of the absence or underdevelopment of the 6th and 7th cranial nerves. In healthy people these nerves control eye and facial movements, such as the smile. At birth, the deficit is often diagnosed when infants cannot suck and may require alternative feeding methods to ensure nutrition. In adulthood, the most noticeable public difference of these folks from the average population is their inability to move their eyes and the lack of a smile.

Cole's interviews with Mobius syndrome individuals reveal much about the relationship between facial movement and interior states of feeling. In one conversation, for example, a man with Mobius remarked, "I have [sic] found it very difficult to communicate feelings throughout my entire life, whether as a child or with my wife, though I think I am getting better at it now. I don't really know how to communicate happiness or sadness."[56] It was only in later life that he realized he could communicate to other people through the use of hand movements signaling that he was glad to see them or that he was enjoying a conversation. He feels that his muted emotional reactions were very helpful in his job as a church minister, where showing a lot of emotion could potentially be counterproductive.

In another interview, Cole brings together a group of children diagnosed with Mobius. He is curious if the children, like the adults he spoke with, also have difficulty expressing emotion. He wonders if they will run around and laugh and play like any group of young playmates or if they will be as immobile and passive as their faces? Research done by Jane Walker with young Mobius patients had previously demonstrated that if the children are shown cards with pictures of different facial expressions, they were unable to pinpoint the feeling that particular person was experiencing.[57] However, Cole's experience being around the children contradicted Walker's findings, at least somewhat. Most parents of the children reported that their kids could indeed read other's facial expressions for affect. Yet, their experiences as parents of children with Mobius did reveal characteristic, and often very challenging, commonalities related to lack of emotional expression. One parent, for example, told a story of her child not sleeping at night for four years. "Thinking back, I realize it was because she couldn't shut her eyes. She may have just woken up and been frightened of the dark and she couldn't shut her eyes."[58] It seems that although the children's parents reported that they could indeed understand the facial expressions of others, these families did have children who exhibited unusual behaviors that ran from the biological to the emotional.

The children themselves spoke of social problems as well. Claire, for example, reported, "I've always felt it difficult to express how I feel. I know it's only in the last couple of years that, say, at church when I meet someone I just say 'I can't smile' and then it becomes easier." Cole speaks of another little boy. "In place of the spontaneous volcanic emotions children experience, display, and learn to control, Duncan, like Clare, inhabits a rather isolated world of deliberation and thought."[59] Their children, at least in his interviews, all had trouble feeling and expressing emotion and they each had difficulty relating with others.

The most consistent link between all the children was the immobility of their faces. Here, a return to Farrer's concern regarding the possibility that face transplant patients might have immobile faces is helpful. Might an immobile transplanted face lead to social misunderstandings akin to individuals with Mobius?

Another debate, this one focused on the potential psychological and social was the suggestion that becoming physically more socially acceptable after a long period of disfigurement can lead to a unique kind of social dilemma. Baker and Smith conducted a study where facially disfigured patients suffered from not only the initial trauma and injury, but also from their lack of coping skills to deal with a more beautiful face than they were used to having.[60] Baker and Smith quote sociologist Erving Goffman's work on how transformations from socially undesirable and unattractive to attractive can completely challenge a "cured" disfigured individual. "The patient is cast adrift from the more or less acceptable protection it has been offered [by the disfigurement] and soon finds, to his surprise and discomfort, that life is not all smooth sailing.[61] If this is true, then the facially disfigured who have become accustomed to not being noticed or looked at in a Goffman-esque "smooth-sailing" fashion must relearn how to be a public figure who is expected to conduct themselves in a stereotyped social manner that most people have learned since birth. Certainly, any face transplant recipients who have lived a long life in the shadows would find a new and even attractive face not the immediate psychological panacea others might expect.

Summerton and Agha have argued that for many the opportunity for a face transplantation surgery would indeed be a life-saving maneuver if only because so many facially disfigured people feel so very depressed and alone. "Face transplantation would indeed be a life altering experience for an individual with facial disfigurement. It could be considered as potentially life-saving by preventing suicide and even life-giving by increasing the individual's participation in society and potentially opening up new opportunities for them such as marriage, a better job, going out to dinner without being stared at or ridiculed."[62] Houston and Bull's study tested whether people in public do indeed look away or avoid folks with disabilities. Up until this empirical study conducted in 1994 there were no published research-based studies that supported these claims. Houston and Bull designed a clever study to test precisely how much passengers on a subway car would avoid a woman in one of four "face" conditions. In the first condition, she used makeup to cover her port-wine stain. In the second condition, her face had her port-wine stain showing. In the third condition, makeup was added to create a narrow scar running down the length of her face. Finally, she was made up to appear with a bruise under one eye. Their results demonstrated that in the port-wine stain condition people chose not to sit next to her more frequently than in any other condition. Her normal discolored face and bruise prompted the least interpersonal distancing. Investigators conclude that "facially disfigured people may not merely be imagining that they were avoided."[63] Other research has suggested that disfigured people waiting to cross a street are avoided by others.[64] Also, people will offer less money and spend less time with disfigured people who work for charities.[65]

Burn victims, and other folks with severe facial trauma, as surmised from the Houston and Bull study, must experience very difficult episodes of social staring and avoidance. In all fairness, we are not exactly a culture awash with role model opportunities. Guides in tempering our encounters with facially disabled folks are few and far between. After all, if our most basic human interactions with another are vis-à-vis their face, then exhibiting discomfort at a missing or severely distorted face is not necessarily an indication of rudeness or insensitivity. Perhaps it should be an expected reaction and understood as very human. Missing here is a creative transition for both the disfigured and nondisfigured. It is informational to examine how one town that did find a method to communicate with others that individuals with facial disfigurements were nearby. After WWI, in the town of Sidcup, England, the benches near the hospital were painted blue. This colored warning alerted visitors around the area of Queen Mary's Hospital that a veteran with a severe facial wound might be sitting. In that way, passersby could prepare themselves for faces ruined by war. This small town courtesy to both wounded resident and visitor is indeed creative and sensitive. It also speaks to deeper and more complex issues related to the difficulty of encountering people with facial traumas.

Changing Faces is a London-based patient advocacy group for facially disfigured persons. The agency has tried to raise public awareness on behalf of the facially disfigured to diminish social shunning. Their take on facial disfigurement is that far more people will have to live with distorted faces than will be able to receive a face transplant. Thus, their stance is that there are two ways to combat the problems faced by those with disfigurements. One way is to educate the public. The Changing Faces Web site offers extensive personal stories and pictures.[66] Everything from facial injuries to facially distorting genetic diseases is featured. The goal is specifically to sensitize others to facial deformity and humanize those who love them. Alternatively, they have also tried to teach those with unusual facial configurations to become more aware of how their behavior may contribute to the public's view of them. One study tested the theory that interpersonal training could improve the social experiences of the facially disfigured. They found that participation in a workshop teaching coping skills yielded many positive results for the participants. One respondent, for example, had difficulties knowing how to answer young children's questions. After training the participant responded that they had learned how to effectively cope with children's queries. Most participants reported a lowering of social anxiety, depression, and social avoidance. The results suggest the possible benefits of teaching and of supporting individuals with facial disfigurements, using this kind of group therapy approach.[67]

When considering the extent of facial injury suffered by Isabelle Dinoire, it is unreasonable to seriously consider that training the public, or even training an individual to cope, would heal the psychological traumas she endured. A *New York Times* article reported that upon return from the hospital Dinoire had to remove the mirrors in her apartment. "She could deal with looking at herself in the mirror when she was prepared, but the unexpected, looming image of herself was too disturbing."[68] Expecting society to somehow adjust with this level of facial trauma is perhaps asking too much. Additionally, training Dinoire to cope with the reactions to others may be beyond the level of her ability. Her condition was devastating—exposed teeth, no nose or chin. Changing Faces came out against face transplantations in favor of supporting the acquisition of coping skills and public education.

In the year before the first face transplantation there were a number of extensive medical debates. The commentaries were about the complex relationships between disabilities, identity, and face transplantation. "Some people affected by facial disfigurements report that their altered facial appearance no longer reflects the 'real me.' The proposed early recipients of face transplants may well prefer the prospect of a normal appearance, however, the effects on self-perception of 'wearing' a face that previously fronted an entirely different identity is entirely unknown. Issues about projecting the 'real me' are likely to remain."[69] It is difficult to anticipate how a face transplant will change a disfigured person's sense of identity. There are many factors to consider. The person's age, gender, and the type of disability or injury they possess are all parts of the identity equation. With so few facial allotransplantations thus far, the best possible guess may be found in the literature on cosmetic surgery. After all, having a surgically created face is, in many ways, not one's own.

THE NOSE OF MYSELF

One way to understand what is at stake in this unknown landscape of face transplantation is to look at plastic surgery. What is known, for example, about receiving the nose of another when it has been surgically shaped? When compared to face transplantation, cosmetic nose jobs and face lifts seem rather blasé. However, in a partial face transplant procedure both the nose and face are transformed in ways that are similar, if not exact, with plastic surgery. In Dinoire's case, of course, her nose, cheeks and chin, and lips were lost and replaced. The literature therefore on nose and face plastic surgery procedures may be helpful in understanding what kinds of psychological effects may be at play after face transplantation.

Marcia K. Goin and John M. Goin report the motivating factors at play in different types of plastic surgery. Their research follows patients who seek out cosmetic changes. They also follow up the postoperative clients and assess their psychological experience. While they state, "it is impossible to make generalizations about the total population of aesthetic facial surgery patients. People of different age groups, sexes, and ethnic groups, and psychological status tend to seek different reasons."[70] Citing Webb's study, they note that plastic surgery patients fall into three categories. There is the "emotionally dependent group, the worker group, and the grief group."[71] The emotionally dependent group was bonded by their "repeated difficulties in meeting adult responsibilities and were very insecure." The second group, the "worker" group, included people who were deeply involved with their careers and friends made at work. The grief group was comprised of people who had experienced the loss of a loved one. Overall, people from these groups "were more likely to be suffering from grief, loneliness, depression and loss."[72] Goin and Goin found that rhinoplasty patients were in general "more psychologically disturbed than the general population."[73] They were as a group "more restless, self-critical, and sensitive to the opinions of others."[74] Face transplant patients do not, of course, chose to receive an allotransplantation procedure under the same conditions as a traditional cosmetic surgery client. However, there is an element of choice in the matter. In the book *Heroes with a Thousand Faces: True Stories of People with Facial Deformities and Their Quest for Acceptance*[75] author Laura Greenwald tells the experiences of individuals who have sustained dramatic facial distortions. One chapter deals specifically with the topic of face transplantation. Gleaned from this section is how choice is involved when deciding about face transplantation. A burn patient, for example, speaks of the desire to correct the texture of her face and to feel normal again. If plastic surgery patients can be split into groups that separate them into "emotional, worker, and grief," then maybe the same categories can be applied to those desiring a face transplant. It is unknown still if seriously pursuing the procedure is related to the same or different motivational factors. Only with more face transplantations can trends be uncovered and analyzed.

Rhinoplasty patients have the distinction of being the only plastic surgery patients to murder their surgeons. Some rhinoplasty patients love their new look, but experience a difficult shifting of their identity. Others hate their new look, but their sense of identity has not been challenged. There is a disruption between the postsurgical esthetic experience and one's personal sense of identity. Depressive mood states and the acting out of negative behaviors have also been reported for nose reconstruction patients. Some rhinoplasty patients, for example, lament the loss of a family resemblance, fearing that they have erased the nose of their father or mother. In a depressive state they may long for their former look. Sander Gilman's book *Making the Body Beautiful* chronicles the history of plastic surgery vis-à-vis the nose reconstruction. Perhaps the most well-known surgeon of the late 1800s was Jacques Joseph, an orthopedic surgeon training under Julius Wolff, one of the leaders helping patients who had noses deformed by syphilis. Joseph firmly believed in the power of the nose job to cure sorrows. He would take pictures of his patients after surgery dancing in a liberated postsurgical mania. Many early corrections of the nose were to erase Jewishness or Blackness or Irishness from one's face—self-chosen ethnic cleansing. Revealed here is how much meaning the shape of one's nose may possess. One, in fact, could mourn a severed connection with one's family and ethnicity—a very real dilemma for rhinoplasty patients.[76]

Facial trauma, of course, separates the face transplant candidate from the cosmetic surgery candidate who typically battles an uncomfortable self-image. Nevertheless, if we listen to face-lift and rhinoplasty patients, they can shed light on possible reactions to receiving a transplanted new nose or face. To a person profoundly disfigured, having any nose must be considered the best case scenario. However, the psychological significance of the nose may be great. Noses may in fact be complicated; Isabelle Dinoire's reaction to her new face is expressed in a remarkable comment about her nose. During a conversation with her family members she casually mentioned that her nose was itchy. She then changed course and said "I have a nose that is itchy." To Dinoire, her nose was not entirely hers—at least not yet. If newly sculpted noses have been noted to cause a disrupted sense of family origin—or even a mixed psychosexual response, then one must consider possible similar effects with facial allografts.

Wearing the nose of another could very well elicit fantasies or concerns of a new ethnic identity. Conceivably, there could be a perceived identity with the family members of the face donor. Whether or not these connections with rhinoplasty patients would be positive or negative, we cannot be sure, but they seem important as a way to understand face transplantations at a deeper psychological level. Face lifts do not translate as neatly to face transplants. Although both procedures involve skin flaps, clearly a tightening of one's own skin versus the application of another's facial skin is vastly different. However, there are certain types of face lifts that involve changing the underlying muscle and bony structure, and these kinds of more radical facial changes have been noted to cause depression and a disrupted sense of identity. It must also be considered that a change of face does not need to be negative—even if it is challenging and disruptive. Carosella and Pradeu have even suggested that the drastic changes inherent with identity shifts can be potentially positive. "The graft of a visible organ can lead to a full expression of one's identity, making the individual aware that to be oneself is to change constantly, and to accept oneself as changing."[77]

There is also the consideration that a new face could in fact be more attractive than the old face. A new face, if carefully concealed with makeup, could bring more positive social attention toward an individual than they have received in the past. When young individuals have had a rhinoplasty, it is not uncommon for them to become tempted with "a variety of new impulses and temptations."[78] This newfound attraction could thrust an allograft recipient into a kind of postadolescent crisis whereby they have to renegotiate their social relationships within established and new relationships.

CHOOSING THE RECIPIENT

In light of these many considerations of how face transplant patients may feel changed and challenged psychologically, choosing the best possible patient is vital. Ironically, the best face transplant candidates may be the ones who do not really want to have one. Many individuals who have survived traumatic facial wounds, burns, or even botched gunshot suicide attempts and have adjusted to their appearances and do not desire the procedure may in fact be the ideal patients. This paradox has been noted by the Working Party of the Royal College of Surgeons of England in a 2007 review of the clinical issues surrounding face transplantation. They conclude, "the more vulnerable will be less well equipped to deal with the aftermath of complex transplant surgery, uncertain outcomes, and ongoing treatment regimens."[79] Furr and colleagues have even recommended that "the transplant candidate should be someone who has not adjusted to disfigurement and has experienced a gross decline in quality of life."[80] Both Peter Butler in England and Maria Siemionow at the Cleveland Clinic have spoken at length about choosing the best patient for the procedure. Oddly, the surgical team that worked on both on Clint Hallam and Isabelle Dinoire did so even though there were indications that they were not the best patients from a psychological perspective. Much has been made of Ms. Dinoire's mental status at the time of the transplant, especially questioning if she was suicidal.[81, 82] When Dinoire was interviewed after the injury she commented, "after a very disturbing week and lots of personal worries, I took drugs to forget."[83] Consequently, critics contended that she would have problems accepting and coping with the stress created by the surgical procedure and the subsequent media exposure.

In an article addressing these issues French transplant surgeon Devauchelle made three points to defend their choice of Ms. Dinoire as their patient. First, the authors argued that "the presumed fragility of a patient" should not deny them "the best therapeutic management." Second, although they neither directly confirm nor deny the fact that Dinoire was suicidal at the time of her transplant, they still state, "would someone's suicide constitute a sign of weakness for certain people, while for others, within a different cultural context, it is a sign of strength or wisdom?"[84] Finally, they remind readers that no one really is in a position to know the details of the patient's life before the facial trauma, but that Dinoire was "attended to over six months by three different teams of psychiatrists. All the experts consulted concluded unanimously that she was in a position to understand the issues of the innovative treatment that was being proposed to her and, subsequently to deal with the constraints of the adjuvant treatment that was being proposed to her...."[85] Clearly, much negativity, both in the popular and academic press called for this very straightforward accounting. Not only had Dinoire's right to the operation been called into question, but also her right to be suicidal at the time of the trauma. Ultimately she was able to still demonstrate wellness of mind to understand the consequences of the decision to have the procedure. Dinoire signed her informed consent form on November 24, 2005. On it she agreed that she "[sic] perfectly understood, all the explanations that were given to me."[86]

HOSPITAL TEAM READINESS

In 2006 the Working Party of the Royal College of Surgeons reported on the "15 minimum requirements to be fulfilled before a unit or institution should contemplate undertaking facial transplantation."[87] For purposes here, the report has been condensed to three main conclusions: 1) the importance of technical competence and medical, social, family, and financial and follow-up care regardless of a positive or negative outcome; 2) the suitability of a patient's physical, psychological, and social attributes; and 3) issues related to informed consent, that is, if it is ethical to put healthy individuals on immunosuppressant drugs for the remainder of their lives to maintain the allograft. Further complicating the situation was that there were no prior cases to inform the patient in the event that the facial graft should fail. The best educated guess was that if the face transplant underwent a complete bout of rejection, the patient would not be much worse than before the transplant. Losing the graft would expose parts of their disfigured faces that had been exposed prior to surgery. Then, traditional replacement procedures would be initiated, such as grafts with the patient's own skin. However, this was just a guess, and no one would really know the outcome of this unfortunate occurrence until it really happened.

FACE TRANSPLANTATION

Before face transplantation could be carried out, some other firsts had to take place. Some barriers in technique had to be overcome. One precursor to the first face allograft was surgeries replacing scalps lost in industrial accidents. Although these kinds of accidents have diminished with increased workplace safety, they still do occur.[88] The first successful replantation of a full scalp avulsion could only occur after the refinement of microsurgery techniques. In 1974 Miller and his colleagues repaired a scalp removed in an industrial accident.[89] Technically speaking, the first facial transplant occurred on September 2004 on a seventy-two-year-old Chinese woman who had a large cancerous tumor removed from the top of her scalp. Instead of using traditional approaches to restoring her skin, such as using much of her own tissue to reconstruct the area, her doctors agreed to try and use a donated flap of skin to cover the back of her scalp as well as two donated ears.[90] The surgery was a success and offered hope to others who had suffered large amounts of tissue after the removal of cancerous scalp tissue.

Restoring not just the scalp but the actual face has been a goal of surgeons whose mantra as reconstructive specialists has always been "replace like with like." However it is virtually impossible to reconstruct many of the face's details in a highly satisfactory manner. After WWI much medical information was published about the challenges associated with fixing faces that had been ravaged by war. "The most horrendous facial wounds came to the clinics of the Allies and the Central powers. Faces were literally blown away, jaws ripped off, and skulls crushed, and soldiers with such wounds lived."[91] Soldiers wounded on the battlefield with facial wounds were marked with a special placard asking that they all be sent to Queen Mary's clinic in Kent, England, for repair. In this way as much work as possible could be performed. The organization of patients by type of injury helped to greatly increase surgical skills for all types of head injuries. Surgical skills at this point in history had advanced to where reconstruction of noses and jaw lines had been performed for cosmetic reasons. Facial restoration of the nose, lips, chin, and cheeks performed after the First World War, making the faces look as they did before the injury was just as challenging then, as it is today. "These were clearly reconstructed faces," reconstructive surgeon Harold Delf Gillies noted twenty years after the war, recalling "the old gibe of the French that 'before' the patient was horrible, and 'afterwards' ridiculous."[92] John Barker's comments from July 2007 do not offer much more hope that advances have been made with helping individuals with disfigured faces look normal again. "We have some patients with 120 operations and you still look at them and it's hard to sit in front of them."[93]

ISABELLE DINOIRE

Isabelle Dinoire's personal story is no less full of controversy and intrigue than Hallam's. A divorced mother of two teenaged girls, she lived in the northern city of Valenciennes, France. According to her doctor on May 28, 2005, Isabelle took a large amount of sleeping pills and became unconscious. While no one besides Dinoire can tell if she was suicidal at the time, she did take enough of the drugs to become so deeply unconscious that she did not notice the family's Labrador retriever pawing and chewing at her face, perhaps in an attempt to revive her. Sadly, when she did awake and tried to light a cigarette, "it wouldn't stay between my lips." She then looked down … "and saw the pool of blood and the dog beside it."[94] Isabelle's face had sustained extensive traumatic loss. After she was rushed by her mother to the emergency room, she was transferred to the cranio-maxillo unit in Amiens where she was examined by Devauchelle, the resident expert in head and face reconstruction, who made an assessment of her injury and determined that it was grim. Medical examination revealed that she had lost the lower half of her nose, "upper and lower lips, the whole chin, and adjacent parts of right and left cheeks. The injury involved all soft tissues of the face down to the skeleton and teeth."[95] It was the reconstructive surgeon's opinion that if traditional means of repair were performed that it would take "at least four or five operations to restore the four missing anatomical units, and would probably have led to poor aesthetic and functional outcomes ... [Thus] composite tissue allotrans-plantation was chosen as the first therapeutic option to reconstruct the patient's face."[96] She was a particularly complicated case that would involve three facial structures that are almost impossible to pleasingly reconstruct. English reconstructive surgeon Peter Butler noted in an interview the challenges of facial reconstruction: "The nose, lips, and chin. These elements are very difficult, if not impossible, to reconstruct adequately using conventional methods."[97] During her first days in the hospital her wound was cleaned. She began a routine of intensive physiotherapy to reduce scar tissue buildup and maintain flexibility to the jaw muscles and muscles responsible for facial expression. Despite ongoing physiotherapy, time was of the essence for Dinoire. Unfortunately, despite efforts otherwise, she continued to develop increasing amounts of scar tissue in the remaining facial muscles. By the time a donor had become available, she could only open her mouth 19 mm—just a tiny crack.

At a psychosocial level she was struggling. Every trip into a public space was a challenge—she even wore a dental surgical mask while going to shower within the hospital. Ventures out of the hospital included the wearing of a mask to shield her missing face. Her experiences in public ran the gamut from feelings of acceptance to mild discomfort to a painful shunning. "Some people don't say anything out of the ordinary; they say hello, they talk. Other people look and shrink back. In the shops, some people even hide out of the way."[98] Meanwhile, Dinoire's doctors were following guidelines from the French National Ethics Committee to gain authorization from various French ethics agencies to harvest the partial face from a dead beating-heart donor. After a six-month wait permission is granted and a suitable donor is found. Dinoire, out on a family day excursion, was called back to the hospital and quickly prepared for surgery. The donor was an excellent match for Dinoire, and the operation occurred early the next morning.

Face Transplant Procedure

The allograft donor was "a brain-dead woman aged forty-six years who died from a severe, irreversible cerebral ischaemia."[99] She was an excellent match for skin, blood type, and antigens. The transplant had to be removed from the donor in the exact shape of Dinoire's injury. To ensure the most accurate cut, a metallic mask was manufactured to the exact shape of the recipient's face. This metallic template pattern was subsequently placed on the donor's face and traced to ensure a perfect match to the dimensions and shape of the injury. Because Dinoire had lost her skin and the underlying fat and muscle, the transplant included the donor's subcutaneous tissue,

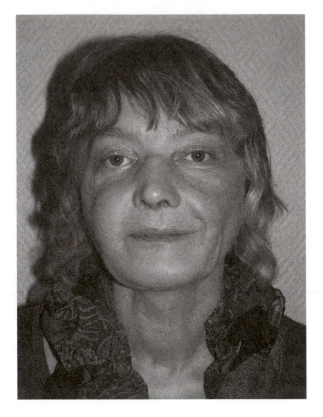

Courtesy of Isabelle Dinoire

cheek fat pads, muscles, and facial nerves. A small flap of skin was removed from the donor's upper left arm. This section of skin would be applied under Dinoire's breast as a sentinel flap. Instead of taking biopsy samples from her face, this little skin flap was used "to monitor indirectly the immunological behavior of the graft, aiming to avoid damage to the reconstructed face by repeated skin biopsies"[100] In addition, bone marrow was taken from the donor. The marrow would later be transferred to Dinoire. The procedure was entirely experimental. It was the first time bone marrow had been transferred to a transplant patient without the usual routine of radiating the recipient's own marrow first. Because there was no bone in the face transplant, the medical team hoped that a direct introduction of marrow would suffice to ward off rejection. Perhaps the introduction of donor marrow and stem cells would provide a lessened immunological response.

Great care was taken to prepare the donor's remains for the family. Her "nose-lips-chin triangle was reconstructed with a colored silicone mask, custom-made inside a plaster cast molded on her face at the beginning of the procedure."[101] In this way the first face transplant donor was laid to rest.

The allograft was prepared in a similar fashion to the first hand transplantation. First, the scar tissue was removed, and nerve endings and blood vessels were exposed and prepared for connection using microsurgery. The transplant was placed onto the recipient's face. The arteries on the right side of the face were connected and the clamp was released. Dinoire's blood quickly infused the transplant and normal color was immediately achieved. Additional facial veins and arteries were sutured. Nerves that control movement of the mouth and facial expressions were connected. Next, muscles were attached and finally subcutaneous tissues and skin. Dinoire's physiotherapy was begun forty-eight hours after surgery and was offered twice daily for the follow-up period.

The patient was placed on a variety of drugs immediately following surgery including the antirejection drugs tacrolimus and mycophenolate mofetil and the anti-inflammatory steroid prednisone. The prednisone was initially given in high doses and then was tapered off to maintenance levels. The frozen donor bone marrow was thawed and given on days 4 and 11 after transplantation. Neurological assessment determined that the first facial skin sensations returned around the upper lip area in about 10 weeks followed by full face sensation in the grafted tissue around week 14. At about this three-to-four month period the inner cheeks also became sensitive. For the first time since the surgery numbing agents had to be used for mouth biopsies. Psychological support was offered daily for the first four weeks and then twice weekly. "Psychologically, the transplant was well tolerated in the immediate post-operative period and its quick integration into the patient's new body image was greatly helped by the fast sensate recovery of its skin surface. At the end of the 12th postoperative week, the patient became able to face the outside world and returned progressively to a normal social life."[102]

As remarkable as the entire face transplant story is, there is a one moment in particular that seems more remarkable and astounding than anything else. Briefly mentioned above, it bears repeating. The surgeons in an article for the academic medical journal *The Lancet* describe "when the clamp was released, [and] the whole composite transplant rapidly achieved a normal color and volume."[103] Later however, in a news report, the surgical team embellished the moment in language more suited for the general public and filled with their pure amazement: "When we wipe the face clean, when it comes back to life and we take off the clamps, what we see is a person resurfacing, a new, restored person, and that's the moment a surgeon stops being a surgeon and becomes a man or woman again and can live through the moment with a human's feelings and everything that stirs within."[104]

LOSS OF FACE

In the event that the graft should indeed fail no one really knows what the consequences would be for Dinoire. "Not much is known about unsuccessful face transplant. It is, however, very probable that the patient will be worse, probably much worse, after the unsuccessful transplant than before the surgery."[105] The 2004 Royal College of Surgeons estimated that a graft loss might occur in 10 percent of recipients within the first year and that a substantial loss of the graft from chronic rejection might be in the 30 to 50 percent range.[106] Reasons for graft failure could include blood circulation not being established or postoperative blood clotting; acute rejection due to a severe immunological reaction that is unresponsive to medicine; or chronic rejection that involves the narrowing of the arterial openings. Before conducting her first face transplantation, Maria Siemionow at Cleveland Clinic had to think carefully about the threat of rejection because she was approved to do a full face transplant and had spoken of helping burn victims who tragically do not have faces and would benefit greatly from the procedure. The problem however with using a burn patient is the question: if the graft should fail, would a burn patient have enough healthy body skin to be used to cover an entire face? She estimates that that it would take about 1,200 cm of skin to cover the neck, scalp, and ears.[107] For Isabelle, however, she was told in her informed consent form that the worst case scenario for her would be a loss of the graft and a return to her previous condition. The consent form also broaches the possibility of psychological rejection. The informed consent form advised her

> of the need for frequent, long term psychological supervision: the experience of transplantees proves that there may be, on the part of the recipient, not only a physiological rejection of the transplanted member or organ, but also a psychological rejection. It was for this reason that the first hand transplantee, being incapable of standing the presence of his transplanted member, eventually had it removed. It is therefore essential that frequent psychological consultation be set in place for a course of several years, with either a psychologist or psychiatrist.[108]

The veiled reference to Clint Hallam is of course very revealing.

Fortunately, in the eighteen-month follow-up published by the *New England Journal of Medicine,* Isabelle Dinoire reportedly was doing very well. She had healed well, could chew and swallow food, and appeared to be pleased with her new face. However, she had to still live with the knowledge that her allograft could be rejected by her body at any time. In addition, a close reading of the medical article shows that she had had many challenges in the previous year and a half. After the surgery, she had to deal with many small and significant setbacks. At eight months, she was successfully operated on for a narrowing of a small duct passageway in her mouth by the back molars. Two episodes of acute rejection occurred on days 18 and 214 after transplantation. These reactions were characterized by the gradual development of redness and swelling on the oral mucosa, the skin graft area of the face, and sentinel flap. Rejection was confirmed by biopsies of the facial skin and the sentinel flap. As scary as these acute rejections sound, it is just a fact that where transplants are concerned some degree of rejection is more or less to be expected. Because of advances in drugs to help immunosuppression, rejection rates in kidney transplants have steadily declined to below 20 percent. Beyond the problems of rejection, two infectious complications occurred. On day 185, a type 1 human herpes simplex virus infection of the lips was confirmed. A few days after treatment a second rejection episode appeared over the cheeks on both the allograft and the patient's own skin and was treated by curettage. While on the first immunosuppressive regimen she experienced a progressive decrease in kidney function that was attributed to her immunosuppressant drug. To correct the situation the drug was changed at month 11 after surgery. Five weeks later she developed acute renal failure and hypertension. After a short break for four days from the immunosuppressant drugs, a brief regime of fresh-frozen plasma was delivered intravenously with high doses of immune globulin, after which there were no further acute rejection episodes. Functionally she was doing very well, had normal heat and cold detection, and could open and completely close her mouth. Although it was slow to recover, at eighteen months she was capable of saying closed lip phonemes such as *P* and *B*. She could smile and finally could express facial emotions such as sadness and joy.[109]

POST DINOIRE

Immediately after the first face transplantation in France a hospital ethics committee in the United Kingdom granted permission to Peter Butler and the team at the Royal Free Hospital in London.[110] In the states, the Cleveland Clinic in Ohio was approved for face transplantation led by reconstructive surgeon Maria Siemionow. On April 2006 in Xian, in the capital of Shaanxi Province in northwest China, a face transplant was performed on a thirty-year-old man who had bear bite.[111] Sadly, it has been reported that Li Guoxing died in his rural home in 2008. The cause of death is still being debated. His Chinese doctors reported that Li had started to take herbal medications instead of his immunosuppressing drugs.[112] In March 2007, a third partial face transplantation was performed by a French team on Pascal Coler, who had suffered since childhood with "Elephant Man's" disease. There was very little publicly available information about Pascal's surgery until *The Lancet* published results in August 2008.[113] The delay was clearly to provide the third face transplant patient some privacy. A request to remain anonymous is understandable considering the intense media pressure placed on the first patient, Isabelle Dinoire. Even Dinoire's informed consent documents could not fully anticipate how intense the media scrutiny would be. Only one very short paragraph is given in her consent form, no more really than a suggestion that she would be protected as much as possible from media scrutiny.

Since the third face transplant, the face transplantation team at the Harvard-affiliated Brigham and Women's Hospital in Boston, Massachusetts, led by reconstructive surgeon Bohdan Pomahac, has been granted permission from the hospital's institutional review board to perform face transplant surgeries. Originally the transplant team decided to only pursue candidates already taking immunosuppressant drugs for kidney transplant procedures. By taking people already on immunosuppressant drugs the team can sidestep the problems inherent in asking an otherwise healthy individual to take the toxic drugs. There has been some recent evidence that the risk for an otherwise physically healthy face transplant patient taking immununosupressant drugs is less in danger from the side effects than a patient who has been suffering the effects of an organ failure.[114] Another rationale of using a kidney transplant patient, versus a heart or lung, is that, if the face transplant in some way interfered with the kidney transplant—at this point this is still speculation—that the patient could always go onto dialysis. Obviously, in lung or heart transplant, patients have fewer options. There are multiple advantages for face transplant recipients who have already received other transplants. For one, these individuals are already on immunosuppressant drugs and are compliant. Pomahac anticipates that his contribution to facial allotransplantation is most likely going to perform what might be called a partial partial face transplant.[115] Instead of the entire face or even the nose-chin-cheek triangle, he may replace a part of the face that is simply very difficult to reconstruct in any pleasing manner. The corner of the lips, for example, are tricky to mimic and if someone's donated lips could be used to replace damaged lips, the result might be functionally and esthetically pleasing. Using patients already receiving immunosuppressant medications allows for more flexibility and can permit a more nuanced approach to the surgery, because the need to justify the use of potentially dangerous drugs is removed from the equation. More recently, Pomahac has discussed the hospital's plans to broaden their scope and include anyone who wants and requires a face transplant surgery.

Face transplantation research is still actively being conducted. Most of the recent work on technique refinements is currently being conducted on human cadaver models.[116, 117] Some research teams are working on answering questions related to esthetics results both from a surgical technique point of view and also from a patient point of view. "A result that is perceived to look like 'someone else,' whether that of the face donor or a third identity, could be psychologically challenging."[118] Much of the research on how much and what kinds of immunosuppressant work had been done at the Cleveland Clinic by Maria Siemionow. Working with animal models, she continued until recently to perform both full and partial face grafts on rodent models and experiments with various levels of drug therapy to prevent episodes of rejection.[119] Clearly, Dr. Siemionow's many years of laboratory practice were her way to build the skills she would require in the complex face transplantation performed at the Cleveland Clinic in late 2008. By replacing facial bones, teeth, upper palate, nose, upper lip, and lower eyelids, Siemionow's team transplanted approximately 80 percent of the recipient's face, making it the closest to a full face transplant to date.

TAKING OFF A FEW FACES

Although originating in the scant dreams of the limits of the human body, the realization of a variety of transplant procedures, short of a full head transplant or even brain transplant, has raised new and interesting questions about not only the role that the body plays in one's existence, but to what extent the body can be altered while still housing a human being. Many of these questions are difficult to frame in light of current and past understandings of the human body, understandings that depend on a view that renders the body as a self-enclosed object. Commentators such as the cultural historian Michel Foucault have suggested that medical procedures and the development of medical knowledge have only served to place the body under the domain of scientific knowledge, turning the body into an object of knowledge through a scientific ordering of it, rather than treating it with an attitude of ambiguity. As Foucault himself says in the chapter "Open Up A Few Corpses" from his landmark *The Birth of the Clinic*:

> at a very early stage historians linked the new medical spirit with discovery of pathological anatomy, which seemed to define it in its essentials, to bear it and overlap it, to form both its most vital expression and its deepest reason; the methods of analysis, the clinical examination, even the reorganization of the schools and hospitals seemed to derive their significance from pathological anatomy.[120]

Through pathological anatomy, Foucault argues, the "medical gaze"[121] (the phrase with which Foucault denotes the desire for order and knowledge he finds endemic to enlightenment science), did its best to scrutinize the human body to the point of coercing it into being an enclosed totality of knowledge. Through a process of ordering and "spatialization"[122] of the body and attaching what the philosopher Gilles Deleuze would refer to as a "regime of signs," doctors and medical technicians were able to affix a certain order to the human body, an order that would supposedly afford control over the human body. Through this process, according to Foucault, pathological anatomy was able to take the force of death and all of its ambiguities in the form of illness and lay claim to it within the domain of knowledge.

The implications of Foucault's argument, that the development of medicine in the form of pathological anatomy coincided historically with a medical "perception" that was interested in opening up the mysteries of the body through rational scrutiny, is accurate in its appraisal as such. However, Foucault's assertion that the operation and development of the medical gaze was deeply linked with a desire to define the body as a rational totality, is perhaps, if not misguided, incomplete in its reading of the development of such a medical gaze. Rather than assuming that the body was taken up as a closed off system by medical sciences, as Foucault implies, it might be worthy to consider the idea that the process of "opening" the body to rational scrutiny was less a move of turning the body into an unequivocal entity of clearly defined limits than a process of imbuing the body with more possibility—however linked this move may have been to enlightenment principles of rationality, as a site of new questions and new reflections on reality.

It is not entirely fair to say that Foucault was wrong in his assessment of the development of modern medical knowledge, but, without the insights that one may glean from the development of modern transplant procedures, his definition of medical perception is incomplete. When taking up the history of transplant procedures, especially in light of face transplants, one uncovers a different strain within Foucault's reading of the history of modern medicine as an extension of enlightenment culture principles.

When the face, the last vestige of an appearance based understanding of identity was shown to be fluid in both its appearance, function, and identity, understanding it as an unchanging entity to which one's existence was anchored also began to develop pores, much like the skin, breathing in new ideas and perspiring concepts that had long suffocated it. Transplant procedures have opened up new connections to and within the body toward new processes of function. Such a process of opening up the bounds of the body is not aimed at asserting control of the body's liminal appendages, but, rather, to unravel inured, stolid, and unmoving ways of conceiving and talking about the body—perspectives that have grown not only from the habits of culture, but the habits of reason as well. Once these habits are stripped, a malleability of an individual that not only makes the "body" a more flexible concept (and not an irrelevant one, as radical antihumanists such as Ray Kurzweil would propound[123]), but makes identity equally transformable begins to emerge through a technological innovation that has little do with controlling the body and even less to do with cheating death.

However, how transplant procedures, and specifically face transplant procedures, finally offer the opportunity to redefine the human body as well as the self and identity as radically open and dynamic entities with constantly shifting boundaries, can only first be gleaned in the long history of transplant procedures. By successfully transplanting the face of one person onto the head of another person, the history of transplant procedures arrives at a point where it has become possible for medicine to not only transform the appearance of a person, but in so doing also to challenge the idea that a person's identity, as enmeshed with appearance, is not a static and unchanging entity; rather, just as the face is able to transform and to take on a new life—as much of the rest of the body is able to—so is one's identity. The presumption that one's identity, or even one's existence, is immediately bound to the biological makeup with which one is born, is a concept that finds no legitimacy with face transplants, and, indeed, is eclipsed by insights born of the impact that the procedure has had on individuals and will have on our society.

But the story of face transplants can only begin with its history. To continue our story, we must move out of the past of face transplants and into its future.

2

Dreaming the Face

In the summer of 1993, a now infamous name was involved with a very strange and scurrilous headline, splashing across every major media news source: Lorena Bobbitt. As legend would have it, after a domestic altercation wherein Lorena Bobbitt was to have been sexually assaulted by her inebriated husband John, Lorena stole away from her bedroom for a glass of water only to be distracted by the glint of a kitchen knife. The event that took place after Lorena noticed the knife, now infamous, was enough to make all of America collectively cringe: she cut off a considerable portion of her passed-out husband's penis. Taking off with the better-half of her less-than-better-half's penis, Lorena drove some distance before launching her husband's penis out a window, landing it in an open field by the highway. Immediately after dispensing of her husband's penis, Lorena called the cops to confess her crime. John had his penis sewn back on, and a nationwide media, tabloid, and satire circus ensued (from headline news coverage to a song parody by Weird Al Yankovic). But the weirdness of the Lorena and John Wayne Bobbitt story was only eclipsed in weirdness by what would later occur to John after surgery—the way their story was molded into bizarre pop-culture associations.

With mounting legal and hospital bills towering over him, Bobbitt attempted to cash in on his new found celebrity, by first forming a band, "The Severed Parts,"[1] and then cashing in on a series of appearances in popular culture. But without a doubt, the strangest part of this story was that John, only a year after his wife had severed his penis, appeared in his first porn film: *John Wayne Bobbitt: Uncut.* Two years after his initial foray into the adult entertainment industry, Bobbitt then appeared in *Frankenpenis*—in so far as the story is concerned, the name says it all. As if acting out the collective curiosity of many people after having his penis cut off and reattached, John displayed that in spite of the reattachment of his penis, he was still a normal, anatomically functioning man. Even with the jocularity with which people regard the Bobbitt case, the name of his second porn film, *Frankenpenis*, nevertheless hints at something that people find difficult to deal with, even in the form of a satire. Here, Bobbitt's recovery, having his penis severed and reattached, was not encountered as normal by most people, but as freakish, monstrous, and grotesque, an association evoked by the title of Bobbitt's second film.

Consider the procedure that Chinese doctors performed on a forty-four-year-old man, the recipient of the world's first penis transplant. What was most interesting about the procedure was that after fourteen days the penis was rejected, not rejected in the way one would expect, with physiological problems arising, but rejected by the Chinese man and his wife after they found themselves unable to bear the thought of him having the penis of another man on his body.[2] The outcome of this story was the most unpredictable part. Physically speaking, the penis had attached well to the man's body and indeed was fully functioning with no clear threat of tissue rejection. One would expect a man who had lost his penis in an accident to gladly accept the opportunity of having a penis again, no matter what the cost, but this didn't seem to be true. As *Slate* writer William Saletan pointed out, "[T]he body didn't reject the tissue; the mind did."[3] Something of a similar mental rejection was also at work in the way the story of the Bobbitts was taken up in popular culture. The fantasy of what occurred with John Wayne and Lorena, which John Wayne later embodied in his short-lived foray into the adult entertainment industry, not only glosses over the violence of the domestic situation that resulted in their horrifying story, it also cowers from engaging with the nature-defying story of John Wayne Bobbitt and the terror it could inspire.

Face transplant procedures have inspired their own strange reception in popular culture and by mass media. It is these fantasies of face transplants in popular culture that not only stand as signs of awe at the progress of science, but also a fear of anything new and innovative. Without first examining the fear of the new that exists within popular fantasies of face transplants, the procedure's radical potential stands to suffer its own sort of "mental rejection" at the hands of popular opinion. To begin to assess where face transplants are with the world today, we must first look at the fantasies, fears, and hopes that they inspire in the minds of popular cultures.

PRACTICING FANTASY

In 1924, Andre Breton guided the surrealist movement with his seminal document referred to as the *Manifesto of Surrealism*. This influential work was in part an expression of Breton's intense respect and admiration for Sigmund Freud and the field of psychoanalysis. Specifically, he remarked how Freud's magnificent book on dream interpretation published in 1900 could link together the creative potential of the unconscious with his own love of art. Breton insisted that psychoanalysis was not limited to medical personnel or psychoanalysts but rather afforded everyone from politicians to artists the opportunity to learn how the dream-like, surreal, nighttime landscape could become a space devoted to deepening knowledge about the human mind. The goal, suggested Breton, was to free oneself from the usual daytime preoccupations of work and reality and enter the unknown, where growth and possibility for artistic rebirth awaited. Artists like Joan Miro and Renee Magritte and surrealist authors such as Louis Aragon and Rene Daumal, along with Breton, adopted the importance of the unconscious mind, the bizarreness of free associations, and intellectual challenges of symbolic interpretation to break through established barriers of convention. Freudian psychoanalysis served the surrealists well and helped them to develop new techniques to liberate art from the customary constraints of making sense. Their creations indeed looked and read as works of a dream. Under the surrealists fantasy itself became a centralized and serious pursuit worthy of study, practice, and execution.

One of the creative exercises utilized by the main European surrealist group in the 1920s was a word game they referred to as Exquisite Corpse. A take-off on an old paper and pencil parlor game called Consequences, Exquisite Corpse was transformed by the Surrealists into a utility to expand the dimensions of written speech and to expose the power of unconscious material—material constantly there, quietly lying under the surface of waking life but just dormant, without a venue of expression. Specifically, they reasoned that by releasing writing from the usual restrictiveness inherent in syntax and grammatical rules—using psychoanalytic tools such as free association—that they could open up their writing to randomness and interpretation, increasing creativity and novelty. Exquisite Corpse, in particular, was perfectly suited to gathering group collective fantasy stories. In its original incarnation group players would fold a piece of

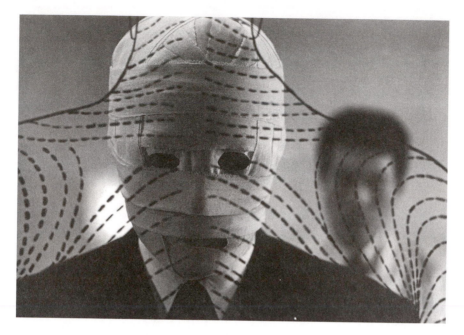

Face of Another. Courtesy of Photofest

paper into four sections, and each player would draw one quarter of a picture on the slip without the others seeing. The game would proceed until the fourth player finished, when at this point the paper was unfolded to reveal a rather surreal-like drawing. Another version of the game was to take a piece of paper and to ask players to generate a line or word and to keep adding to the story with only the benefit of the last line showing to guide a response. As one can imagine, stories written in this way are often filled with strange and unusual segues and associations. In many ways, the game helped to provide the surrealists with the kind of freedom from convention that they desired, and something they further developed in their own work.

PRACTICING FANTASY

In the spirit of Exquisite Corpse, 200 undergraduate college students within three different psychology classes were asked to participate in a classroom teaching exercise about the unconscious and its relationship to fantasy. The students were given instruction on how to create the collaborative story and were informed that they would be writing on the topic of face transplantation. To begin, students were instructed to write the following sentence at the head of a blank piece of paper: On November 27, 2005, doctors performed the world's first partial face transplant on a French woman, Isabelle Dinoire. After she left the hospital.... Once the first line was established, students were instructed to complete the sentence and pass the paper along to another student. Each student would then add their ideas and carefully fold down the paper, accordion style, so that only their last response was showing. The exchanges went on until the sixth turn, when the students were asked to write the last line of the story. After one final exchange, primarily as an act to preserve anonymity, students were asked to open and read the stories to themselves. The narratives were then utilized during class to discuss unconscious associations with face transplantation and to instruct the class on related topics such as free association and symbolic interpretation.

There are numerous ways to analyze the resultant narratives. One approach, for example, would be to concentrate solely on their first impressions, that is, the first recorded sentences. The benefits of this approach include providing an equal level of comparison. A first line-to-first-line comparison across all the stories, for example, permits a balance in the analysis where material related to first thoughts and impressions can be analyzed. However, the weakness here is similar to the first card of the Rorschach inkblot in that caution has to be given for initial responses because the participant could be trying to inject a correct answer, or the best response, instead giving a less-monitored contribution. As students sitting in a traditional classroom setting, they were in a rather singular mode of expression leaning toward the scholarly and intellectual—what Freud referred to as secondary process. People who are administered the inkblot, for example, often give stilted replies that they think the test administrator expects them to utter to appear mentally healthy, or intelligent, and so forth. Thus, in order to expose less-censored replies in a free associative writing exercise, it is important to forgo this first impression method.

An alternative method to analyze the collective stories is to use one whereby the entire story that is categorized, i.e., a violent story, has its merits by offering a glimpse of what the entire narrative may mean. However, it is very difficult to really get a sense of how to organize all the materials, because they are coming from many different authors, into a cohesive thematic narrative. Another approach would be to analyze them as one does in a psychodynamic dream interpretation. Here, the analysis might proceed by locating where the feeling state begins, such as fearful if it is written that the face is falling off, and then tracing the evolution of the storyline toward, perhaps, a more positive or more negative feeling state.

The strength of this approach is its ability to see what kinds of first impressions appear and if and how the stories find resolution or escalation in the themes raised. Stories that begin rather negatively, filled with fear or blood, might resolve themselves later on toward more positive states such as hope. This progression might hint that, although the fantasies related to face transplantation are initially psychically challenging, they can be overcome and accepted by the subjects, and ergo, ourselves upon further exposure. Or, the stories might turn less positive as the stories grow, suggesting that the topic of face transplantation becomes more uncomfortable for the students.

Ultimately, for our purposes here, a method was chosen that would best describe each of the responses emitted. Because this was the first qualitative study conducted on face transplantation, special care was needed to take from the data as much as possible. The rationale became to explore the responses in such a way that would reveal as much as possible about what happened during the writing exercise. It was decided that an exhaustive count of the different topics raised would most accurately achieve that goal. Thus, a content analysis approach was used whereby each line of the stories was analyzed for its thematic content. Each theme was identified, quantified, categorized with like themes, and finally analyzed for precisely the kinds of fantasies that emerge about face transplantation.

RESULTS

Thirty-six different themes were identified for a total of 250 coded responses. The themes themselves ranged from the most frequently mentioned—celebrity/comic book characters—to the lowest level of responses. For example, there was only one mention across all stories for knives. Themes were organized into three categories. If a topic was mentioned more than thirteen times, it was placed in the most frequent response category, less than thirteen but more than five it was placed in the middle response category, and any mentions less than five was placed in the category labeled low frequency.

HIGH-FREQUENCY RESPONSES

High-frequency responses comprised 53.2 percent of the total number of responses coded. The category includes the following topics: celebrity/comics, food, face slipping off/defective/rejection, animals, violence, and finally, masks/Halloween/makeup.

Celebrities/Comics (12.4 Percent of Total)

Thirty-one of the responses, making up 12.4 percent of the data, included references to famous celebrities or comic book characters. An example of such a comment is: "She realized that Bob Barker had the same surgery. Her heart sank as she realized she was not the only one with a face transplant."

Food (12 Percent of Total)

Thirty of the responses mentioned food and liquids, comprising 12 percent of the total comments counted. For example, "After she left the hospital, she wanted ice cream."

Face Slipping Off/Defective/Rejection (10.4 Percent of Total)

Twenty-six mentions of the facial allograft becoming rejected or slipping off were recorded, making up 10.4 percent of the total. Two examples of these comments in the narratives are: "After she left the hospital, her face fell off" and "Her immune system was rejecting the transplant, her face was rotting."

Animals (7.2 Percent of Total)

Animals were quite notable with eighteen mentions in the narratives, making up 7.2 percent of the total responses coded. An example is: "Unfortunately, seconds later Isabelle was bitten by a poisonous centipede and died immediately."

Violence (6 Percent of Total)

It was not uncommon for the stories to include violence. Violent themes emerged fifteen times in the narratives, comprising 6 percent of the total. For example, "She got so drunk she lost her car and was mugged and raped. The police found her body three weeks later."

Masks/Halloween/Makeup (5.2 Percent of Total)

Masks being worn by themselves or combined with Halloween and makeup comprised thirteen of the comments for a total of 5.2 percent overall. For example, "She thought the lady was dressed up for Halloween, she looked so scary."

MIDDLE-FREQUENCY RESPONSES

Middle-frequency responses comprised 32.4 percent of the total number of responses coded. The category includes the following topics: unattractiveness, beauty, sex/gender change, sexuality, doctor incompetence, being unrecognizable, pain, husband/family, fear, being laughed at, and finally, mentions of sports.

Unattractiveness (4.4 Percent of Total)

Concerns of being unattractive and becoming ugly through the face transplant procedure were mentioned eleven times in the stories, making up 4.4 percent of total comments coded. An example of such a comment is: "She looked in the mirror and decided she was still ugly on the inside."

Beauty (4 Percent of Total)

The beauty of the transplant itself was expressed ten times in the narratives, making them 4 percent of the total. An example of beauty in the stories is: "The transplant was so beautiful!"

Sex/Gender Change (3.6 Percent of Total)

There were nine comments related to sex and or gender changes in light of the face transplantation, making up 3.6 percent of the total. For example: "But many confused her as transsexual and her career began to suffer."

Sexuality (3.2 Percent of Total)

Eight mentions of a sexual nature were made in the collective stories, comprising 3.2 percent of the total comments. An example of a comment related to sexuality is: "She decided that this made her too horny, so she had to stop."

Doctor Incompetence (3.2 Percent of Total)

Eight comments were made expressing concerns with doctor incompetence after the face transplant operation, making up 3.2 percent of the total number of responses coded. For example, "She then sued the doctor because of her awful appearance and his malpractice and won 20 million dollars in a settlement."

Being Unrecognizable (2.8 Percent of Total)

Comments about becoming unrecognizable made up 2.8 percent with seven statements counted. For example, "Her family realized they took home the wrong person since she was all bandaged up."

Pain (2.8 Percent of Total)

Pain was mentioned seven times in the collective stories, making up 2.8 percent of the comments coded in the study. "She was in pain for 13 days" is an example of this type of statement.

Husband/Children (2.4 Percent of Total)

Six examples of the words husband or children were counted in the sample, making up only 2.4 percent of the total. For example: "In the morning, she made breakfast for her husband and two children."

Fear (2 Percent of Total), Being Laughed at (2 Percent of Total), Sports (2 Percent of Total)

Each topic appeared five times in the narratives, for a total of 6 percent. For example, "The doctors laughed in her face (that wasn't hers)."

LOW-FREQUENCY RESPONSES

Low-frequency responses comprised 14.4 percent of the total number of responses coded. Many of the topics here received only one mention. The category includes the following topics: blood, vomit/gas/urine, pain medication, media attention, space aliens, plastic surgery, recovery, surgery, scars, smell, insanity, death, mirror, religion, crimes, knives, inside/outside, needing help, and finally mothers.

Blood (1.6 Percent of Total)

There were four mentions of blood. An example of this is: "Her face was bleeding so much, people were lined up outside the hospital to donate blood." Only 1.6 percent of the responses were about blood.

Vomit/Gas/Urine (1.6 Percent of Total)

There were also four mentions of other types of bodily fluids. "After eating, she got really sick and started to barf all over herself." This category only represented 1.6 percent of the total number.

Pain Medication (1.2 Percent of Total)

Although a small total percentage-wise at 1.2 percent, there were three comments pertaining to pain medications. For example, "Within weeks she was addicted to oxycontin, the popular painkiller."

Media Attention (1.2 Percent of Total)

Only three students mentioned the media, for another total of 1.2 percent. "She took her dog for a walk and the paparazzi took her picture."

Space Aliens (1.2 Percent of Total)

Likewise, only three comments were about space aliens, for a very small 1.2 percent of the total responses. For example, "Then the space alien crossed the street."

Each of the following categories received two or fewer mentions in the narratives. Each topic comprised less than 1 percent of the total statements coded in the study. This list includes the following: plastic surgery, 2; recovery, 2; surgery, 3; scars, 2; smell, 1; insanity, 1; mirrors, 1; death, 1; religion, 1; crime, 1; knives, 1; inside/outside, 1; needing help, 1; and finally, mothers, 1.

ANALYSIS

The fantasy material is a rich source of uncensored responses about face transplantation. An analysis of the content can provide a kind of map of the unconscious highlighting areas of the unconscious mind activated during the collective story writing exercise. Although not directly asked for the purposes of the classroom exercise, when the students were informally asked after the writing experience, they admitted that they had never heard of Isabelle Dinoire's face transplantation. A few of the students admitted that they had been introduced to the topic of face transplantation, but upon further questioning it was revealed that they had only very superficial knowledge and only some vague notions of the story from the news media. A framework for the narratives has been provided by dividing them into four thematic categories: 1) boundary, 2) the grotesque, 3) identity, and 4) animals.

BOUNDARY

Violations and recognition of boundaries between self and others are present in the data. Asking people to free associate about face transplantation raises many connections to boundaries and boundary violations. When presented with the term "face transplant," a variety of comments emerge concerning unconscious anxieties about mixing body parts, concerns of merging perhaps uncontrollably with others, and even violent encounters and punctuations of our physical boundaries. Based on these fears of boundary loss and penetration, it can be suggested that the removal and subsequent replacement of another person's face for one's own breaks one of our most fundamental psychological boundaries, that is, that we exist as separate entities from one another. By challenging the security of this assumption all types of anxieties pour forth in the narratives.

The most common forms of the boundary violations, for example, can be found in the frequent mentions of food, animals, violence, sexuality, and space aliens/geographic violations. Other comments within the realm of boundary include the pain associated with the violation of the surgery and mentions of scars as evidence of the physical violation of one's boundaries. In the stories food played a surprisingly prominent role. Psychoanalyst Michael Eigen proposed in his book *The Psychoanalytic Mystic* that the mouth itself carries with it a heavy psychic load. "It would be a world without a digestive system as we know it. We speak through our mouths, not noses. Speaking is weighted by a background of finding (the right word, prey, food), biting, chewing, swallowing, absorbing. Digestion–respiration follow an in–out mode. Starving–suffocation are primal dreads."[4] Without lips and cheeks Dinoire experienced a crisis not only of physical scarring but also scarring of her psyche.[5] The high incidence of food in the stories may represent anxieties related to getting a transplanted face that cannot successfully service the self in the life-preserving act of ingesting food, its life force. With the usual routes to nourishment missing, malformed, or mismatched to the extent they are not reliable, unconscious fears of starvation and the accompanying more psychological fears of emotional neglect creep in. When surgeon Dubernard first saw her, he commented that she could not even chew and keep food in her mouth. In part, it was this brutal observation that moved him to help her with the transplantation. Since the operation, almost as a way to confirm both her conscious and unconscious fears she was preoperatively coping with, Isabelle herself has spoken about the joys of being able to eat normally again. "I am eating as much as I can.... I love fresh strawberries, but have also eaten omelets, chocolate cake and all kinds of other food, including the odd glass of red wine."[6] Her doctors commented "she certainly does not look like the living dead. She's eating and drinking without dribbling."[7] Her reestablished ability to eat and enjoy food once again pushed the primal survival fears Eigen mentions into the background of her psyche. Nonetheless, about two years after the surgery Dinoire commented that one of the most disturbing aspects of her new face was the feeling of someone else's inner cheeks inside of her mouth. The interior, chewing, digesting part of her mouth now provides her nourishment and simultaneously reminds her that the gift of a transplanted mouth comes with the condition that survival supersedes the disturbing fact that one's mouth is not entirely one's own.

It was not anticipated that there would such a high frequency of responses related to animals in the collective stories. Especially because the students, but for a few, admitted that they were not familiar with how Ms. Dinoire lost her facial skin, it is surprising to find eighteen mentions. One approach to understanding their presence and significance is to hold the collective story results up against the very numerous mentions of Isabelle's dog's behavior while she slept in a highly drugged state. Newspaper reports of the dog's behavior on that night nearly universally conclude the most negative depictions of the dog's intentions. It must be said that it is entirely possible that the dog was gentle, but trying to revive her in a very desperate way. One doctor commented that Dinoire would have to have had a very significant amount of sedating drugs in her system not to feel the effects commensurate with her wounds. Most pet owners would understand that a pet could very well possibly respond to irregular breathing or choking in some responsive way, whether barking or even pawing at the piece of the body that seems to be functioning defectively—in this case her face. Nevertheless, the news media comments ranged from the mild side of aggression, such as statements that the dog "scratched and bit,"[8] to the clearly more distempered, that is, that the "dog chewed her face,"[9] "ripped [her face] from head,"[10] "severely disfigured in an attack by a dog,"[11] "severely bitten,"[12] "savaged,"[13] and "mauled."[14] Reading these descriptions leads to thoughts about why the dog, a Labrador retriever said to be a beloved pet by Dinoire's family, did what it did. In other words, why indeed does the dog seemingly have to be portrayed in such a negative light?

Clearly Ms. Dinoire has to be completely mauled in these fantasy depictions of what happened that night, but why is that so? What purpose do the fantasies serve, and how are they connected to the numerous animal mentions in the collective stories? Certainly at one level the dog and animal references expose anxieties related to a fragile separation or boundary between what is animal, what is human, and what is maybe even both. This concept is explored more thoroughly in the section below.

A second way to understand the confusion over the role the dog played was to have to accept that even beloved pets are indeed, even if trying to be helpful, ultimately animal at nature. In other words, even the most human of dogs are animal. The dog attack brings to the surface unconscious worries that our pets are in fact wild at many levels. It is possible that this forced recognition deeply disturbs some fundamental need to keep at bay the unpredictable and chaotic sides of life. A French dog expert was reported to say that although the dog was helping her by scratching her face that ultimately dogs are carnivores and he was just doing what comes naturally when he chewed off portions of her lips, chin, cheeks, and nose.[15]

A third way to understand the fantasies is to see them as indicators of unconscious fears related to forestall the grisly awareness that we are all quite fragile. Yet, there is a gnawing insistence at a fantasy level that it would take a heinous and wild act of viciousness to dismantle Dinoire's face in this grotesque way. However, it is an obvious fact that our skin barrier/boundary between ourselves and the outer world is indeed very thin and vulnerable. Yet to become conscious of this fragility would cause quite a lot of anxiety and in fact a healthy denial of it is probably what keeps us able to engage in the world outside of our own skins in any meaningful way, either at work or in play. Simply put, human skin is highly vulnerable. There are always at work psychological defense mechanisms preventing the realization of how incredibly vulnerable we are to outside forces. Paper cuts are deeply disturbing for this very reason. The small wound presents us with the irony that something as harmless looking as a piece of paper can cause such a bloody mess, and it is simply deeply disturbing to us. After all, think of the fuss that is usually made after such a cut, showing it to others, making pronouncements that we are bleeding from a paper cut and so forth. Paper cuts expose the horror inherent with having typically human thin skin. Thus, the dog "mauling" reports are in a way necessary to hide awareness that our boundaries between our insides and our outsides are so narrow, that we are so entirely vulnerable to disrepair. If the dog was indeed being gentle and trying to revive an unconscious Isabelle, then that would challenge our beliefs that our skin is reliably protective.

Although there were only three mentions of space aliens, it also is tempting to consider this response in light of the topic of boundary violations. It is not uncommon for people who believe they have been abducted by space aliens to speak of being violated sexually by the abductees. Harvard psychologist John Mack[16] began to work with people who believed that they had been adducted by aliens precisely because of the incredible uniformity of their stories, including that they had experienced various kinds of genital sexual and anal probing.[17] So, maybe the mention of space aliens works at the level of a sexual violation in the unconscious. There is however another way to understand the encounters with space aliens in the narratives. Space aliens can also conjure up fears of geographical boundary transgressions; in the most literal fantasy, for example, is the fantasy that aliens will visit planet Earth and steal our precious natural resources.[18] The connection to Dinoire's facial allograft procedure is somewhat oblique, but compelling. Consider one of the most unusual comments made by a reporter after Ms. Dinoire was first presented to the public during a news conference with her doctors. "Ms. Dinoire's [smile] is a bit crooked, with one side slightly higher and one eye more open. But it is not unlike that of a typical Frenchwoman trying to convey a vaguely insouciant sarcasm, with hints of mordant wit and a certain je ne sais quoi."[19] The comment is both humorous and helps to open up this alternative take on boundaries. The face becomes a place of "Frenchness," the transplanted face a typical French woman's look. Could a non-French woman carry the same look and live in her own country, or does the facial allograft possess a boundary of its own? Does the transplanted face possess its own special facial characteristics that do not translate well beyond France? Perhaps face transplants represent at some unconscious level a kind of recolonization of the face, perhaps an amusing interpretation, but certainly speaks to how nuanced fantasy can be when face transplantations are involved.

THE GROTESQUE

Face transplantation appears to awaken deep fears about becoming or appearing grotesque. Masks and fears of hideous forms abound in the data, suggesting that when asked to think about facial allotransplantation that lying just under the surface are deep fears that we, like Dinoire, could become transformed into someone beastly or grossly disfigured. Clearly, free associating about face transplantation evokes images of both the real threats of receiving a face transplantation, implying that the face could in fact undergo a period of rejection and have to be removed, and at a deeper more unconscious level fantasies of the grotesque that challenge some of the more fundamental beliefs about ourselves as being a whole, undamaged, and a fit container for all the precious goods within. The fear that our face should fall off and reveal the horror of the underside is another way to express a human fear of being exposed to our less-desired human qualities such as vulnerability and the fantasy that we are covered and protected by our thin exterior coating of skin. Also, the fantasy of exposure of the underlying tissue as disfigured and terrifying exposes our human fears that we are not composed of all good, but that in fact bad parts are just lingering under our surface.

Many of the fantasies were about masks and Halloween as kinds of covers over some of our less wonderful human aspects such as, rage, hate, and even inappropriate sexual and murderous impulses. Halloween masks, of course, permit a temporary showing of our less-civilized human impulses in a socially sanctioned holiday spirit. The fun of the scary mask evaporates after the holiday if worn in public, becoming the fodder for most horror films: encounters with masked others on dark nights. That our own face may become the one that is mask-like, as when one has undergone a face transplantation, leads to anxieties that we would become the grotesque figure permanently.[20] Many films have explored this fear of one's face becoming horrific and the subsequent need to deal with other's glances and even one's own facial reflection. In George Cukor's film *A Woman's Face,* Joan Crawford's character Anna Holm's face is disfigured by a scar. She hates her face so intensely that she refuses to hang mirrors in her house.

Intense fears of becoming grotesque are related to many of the other collective story fantasies, such as fears of becoming unattractive and then being laughed at. Isabelle Dinoire wanted her new face, at least in part, to blend in and not scare others away. The third face transplant recipient Pascal Coler literally lived the life of a grotesque figure until French surgeon Laurent Lantieri performed his allotransplantation. A genetic disease caused Coler's face to become covered with large bulbous tumors that distorted his features to such an extent that since the age of six he increasingly had to stay at home. "There were awful times. People would not just stop and stare, some could not bear to be near me. I became a recluse."[21] Justified or not, concerns about becoming unattractive or hideous plague us all at some level and one symptom of that fear is to distance ourselves from those who outwardly manifest our inner terrors. We all learn or at least are introduced to early in life the fact that surface beauty is not important and that we must let our beauty shine from beneath our surfaces. Yet, all cultures still rely on some kind of beauty standard. There are competing views as to what makes one kind of face objectively more attractive than another. Research has suggested that faces judged to be symmetrical are often judged by independent viewers to be the most attractive. Facial symmetry has been linked to a coded genetic message that implies to observers the presence of physical health and fertility.[22] Regardless of why we prefer some kinds of faces over others and rate them as more attractive, ultimately all faces attract an other, but only a certain percentage of faces are considered to uphold the most perfect kind of face. Because only a small fraction of the general public possesses that facial look, it creates a kind of anxiety for everyone else. A fear that one is not attractive enough and worthy enough to garner many of the most basic human needs such as love and companionship becomes a nagging fear. Our faces and how we feel about them therefore become a kind of measure of self-worth. Face transplantations highlight a fear of unattractiveness, that not only could we become grossly disfigured and unlovable, but that we could become ugly by someone else's face put in place of our own, A kind of fear of facial contamination whereby another's not so attractive face is forced onto one's own and then having to cope with the ensuing ridicule and fears that one has become grotesque.

After news of the first allograft had spread in the print and electronic news media one conversation in particular was striking. In a day spa many prevailing fantasies about the healing of the grotesque were being discussed. However, it was not the grotesque per se specifically under discussion that day, but rather evidence that a kind of healing, yet obviously greedy fantasy for the stereotyped face of beauty. "Sure, if my face were injured or disfigured, I would think about a transplant," Ms. Murray said, adding matter-of-factly, that under such radical conditions she would trade her face for a comelier model, one with, say, the vulcanized features of Angelina Jolie.

Why not? Ms. Murray mused. "If celebrities put up their faces for auction after they died, people would be bidding on her features all the time."[23] Others were not so entirely sure. "Replacing your features with those of a donor just to make yourself prettier—that idea is abhorrent."[24] It may in fact be abhorrent, but it is also the ultimate antigrotesque cure.

IDENTITY

Identity issues are highly present in the data. The collective story material clearly suggests that participants were working on issues related to identity when writing the group accounts. Face transplantation appears to tap into anxieties about who we are, how that identity is derived, and where it goes if one's face is lost and replaced with another's. One of the more prominent fantasies overall involved the weaving in of celebrity figures, both those from television and film as well as pulp literature, such as comic book characters.

In fact, celebrities and comic book figures counted as the most mentioned overall fantasy. There are a number of ways to understand the cast of famous figures. First, face transplantation must evoke a doubt about authenticity, that is, does the new face work more as a Hollywood mask, where the real individual is hidden behind a part being played out on the screen, where true identities are never really revealed? Or maybe celebrities emerge in the stories as a kind of famous person stalking fantasy. This fantasy has indeed been expressed. Salon.com's story about face transplantation was one of the few that explored the public's possible reactions, albeit fantasy reactions, to face transplantation. "Will the famous faces of celebrity donors become available? Will crazed fans deliberately deface themselves on the slim hope of getting their idol's face?[25]

Face transplantation triggers celebrity fantasies precisely because people associate celebrity with a kind of greedy masking. We both abhor and are fascinated by the faces of the celebrity figure. Popular culture is awash with the faces of the famous because these faces both remind us of how we look and how we at some basic narcissistic level want to be like them, i.e., rich, loved, and coveted and leading a seemingly flawless existence. Just the very term "face transplantation" is enough to release desires usually approached in a more sublimated or culturally appropriate form, such as *People* magazine or the television tabloid show *Entertainment Tonight,* where we can observe our fantasies as channeled through another's creation, maybe the Fox network or the print media.

Fantasies of the famous also assist us to deal with fears that we are always just a mask and never an authentic being. Carl Jung, a follower of

Freud and a brilliant theorist in his own right, developed the notion of persona or mask. The mask or persona for Jung represented an archetype of self, which acts to shield the person from the more intimate and more unknowable inner world that he called the shadow. The shadow must stay capped. The penalty to release the inner core is to unleash a force of inner self with all the incumbent good and bad aspects of oneself, creating a psychotic whirlwind. The mask, or persona, is the face that the public deals with and the center of one's identity. Although the mask ages and changes, it is constant in its ability to protect our more shadowy parts. When considered in this Jungian framework, celebrities are simply our most direct route to explore the persona/shadow dialectic. The famous represent the mask in its most culturally available form. Face transplantation evokes the resultant loss of persona, and for our culture one's persona is packaged and embodied in the likes of Angelina Jolie and Britney Spears.

Beyond Jung's conceptualization of persona he developed his theory of archetype. For Jung an archetype is the part of our personality connected to all that has come before it in the form of cultural images. We possess a type of genetically inherited set of archetypes that Jung believed connected all humans throughout time to one another. Similar archetypes, noted Jung, across all cultures across history have emerged independent of one another. For example, "the Goddess," "hostile brother," "mother," and even war images/archetypes such as the "mushroom cloud" have always been a part of human experience. It is human nature to project these ancient internal archetypes outside of ourselves either by manufacturing them through art or technology or by placing them upon others among us. Many famous individuals, maybe all wildly famous people, are projections of Jungian archetypes. The most archetypal celebrities may in fact be those who are rumored to have never died; their very existence is dependent on our externalized archetypal projections. Hitler as hostile brother has been rumored to live in Miami Beach; Goddess Marilyn Monroe's death is always called into doubt, as is the authenticity of "seductive son" Elvis's demise. The more undead, the more archetypal, they really are living out our collective projective fantasies rather than who they really actually were in real life. Marilyn Monroe's real life of a depressed substance abuser, suicidal Norma Jean is cloaked by collective projections of a sexually daunting and seductive love goddess. Her real-life woes come as a surprise because the real Marilyn is never known; only the archetypal role she plays out in front of our archetype-hungry eyes. Even her death is not enough to kill off our insistence that she is still alive, because archetypes never cease being. Much rumor was made of Heath Ledger's death at a time when he played an on-screen potent hostile brother archetype. Tabloids have played with the idea that playing the villain drove him to insanity and self-destruction. However, this is not the way to understand his death; only his real-life experiences could illuminate his self-destructive fantasies and behavior. His movie archetype masqueraded his worldly life at a time when he fulfilled an archetypal demand for the masses. Only time will tell if he too joins the undead ranks of celebrities, solidifying his role as cultural archetype. Certainly, winning an Academy Award after his death is a step in the right direction, so to speak.

In this way, the interchangeability of comic book heroes and villains with "real" Hollywood people is more understandable. As archetypes there really is not much difference because both incarnations are not really about characters, but archetypes. Face transplantation, at the level of fantasy, may in fact already be an archetype. It could be that removing one's face is an archetype of unmasking available in many different cultural forms ranging from ancient plays to the comic Scooby-Doo. Related to identity as ever malleable and plastic, face transplantations evoke celebrity archetypes as a way to capture this fundamental aspect of being human—that our identities are flexible and fluid.

Another way to grapple with the undead archetype is to consider the fantasy material that was generated by the popular media, that is, nonmedical literature, about the face transplant donor. The facial skin donor for Isabelle Dinoire was taken from a forty-six-year-old stroke victim, who according to the surgical report in *The Lancet* died from a stroke. However, different versions of the donor's death have emerged, with suicide as the most commonly cited cause of death. Here the donor's face is fantasized to emerge from the dead/undead. The fantasy that the donor committed suicide supports the fantasy that the donor was more "dead" than from any version of natural demise. If she committed suicide, the death would be purposeful and cancel out the random natural cause of death, especially for a person still relatively young at forty-six years old. Suicide makes the donation more acceptable by allowing one to believe that the donor wanted death and that the use of her facial skin to reconstruct the face of another makes the death more palatable; after all, the donor clearly was finished with her face and with full intent was ready to give it up.

Our fears of being harvested for our facial tissue must be indeed very complex and deeply disturbing. Is it possible that our faces could become looted and used against our consent? Suicide seems to be a kind of consent letter to the recipient: the message "I choose not to have this face and therefore it is up for grabs for someone better than I to receive it." Without the suicide fantasy everyone who learns about the transplant would have to always wonder, even if it was at some unconscious fantasy level, if the donor was robbed and brought back to life as an unwilling undead reincarnation—clearly a terrifying prospect. Without a signed letter of consent in hand a chance is taken that the face was taken and recycled in this innovative way without permission. Identity theft here is at its most psychologically painful. Perhaps one day we will all be asked to place a special sticker on our driver's licenses that notifies medical authorities that we do indeed want to be a facial allograft donor, but, until that day, it would not be surprising if this donor suicide fantasy plays a very powerful and necessary role. Identity transfer is cancelled out if the cause of death is suicide and permission to imbue the face with a new identity emerges.

The number of responses in the sex/gender change category differs from the sexuality responses mentioned earlier. Here the respondents were expressing fantasies toward face transplantation that speak to concerns that one's actual gender identification would change with the wearing of someone else's face. It is not clear if the story writers were releasing some unconscious concerns that one's face is the center of one's gender identification and if the face is removed that this basic sense that one is either male or female is disrupted. Nevertheless indeed this could be the case. Losing the face becomes a form of castration where one becomes gender confused. Freud described a case he treated where there was a displacement from the lower body to the upper body. For example, repressed anxieties about touching one's genitals could become expressed in the form of a facial tic. If a psychoanalytic cure is induced, the facial tic is cured by uncovering the repressed sexual guilt. "Where the id is there shall the ego be" said Freud. That is, through psychoanalytic treatment materials deeply hidden within the psyche are brought into the light of conscious thought and rational exposure. As difficult as the processes may be, the once repressed and guilt ridden material becomes healed, and the associated symptom dissolves.

In the collective stories face transplantation seems to evoke a displacement from the upper to the lower. Anxieties related to the loss of a face can perhaps be expressed as a loss of genitals. In Freud's scenario, the patient would displace lower to upper because it was the genitals that caused such great stress and the face that could safely express neurotic energy. It is possible that the more historically accurate statement is to suggest that the face is the greater cause of anxiety in the early twenty-first century than the genitals did in the twentieth. The face has become mapped with highly erotic functions and the proposed castration of face causes a displacement to the genitals. This of course suggests that it has become psychically easier to deal with the loss of the genitals than the loss of a face and we may or may not be willing to make this rather bold conclusion.

An alternative approach is to suggest that by becoming sexual we garner an identity both by identifying with our sexual desires, but also through becoming sexually desirable to others. With face removed, we fear that we have become hideous to others and that we have fallen out of the framework where we had been esthetically pleasing. By losing our sexual identity we experience a loss of self. The face and the genitals are joined in a duet of pleasure identification.

One of the lingering mysteries of Dinoire has been her nonstop addiction to nicotine. "I never stopped smoking."[26] Dinoire was clearly apologetic about the initiation of smoking so soon after the surgery, but nevertheless by doing so she reinserted herself into her own framework of desire. With the act of smoking cigarettes, her needs and pleasure were reinstated into her life: a gift of her new face and resexualization. Even her doctors have had to acknowledge that her choice to smoke was driven by a desire for pleasure. "Her return to smoking is not the best thing. But that's what she wants to do—we can't stop her."[27] Ultimately it is what she wants and needs to feel herself again. Here, the view is that her smoking is not entirely bad, but rather an indication that she is in fact displaying behavior consistent with someone who is engaged in deriving pleasure. Surgeon Peter Butler made the following statement. "I said, well actually, smoking doesn't really interfere with the healing, only early on. She must be getting a lip seal. Isn't that wonderful? You have to be able to make it into a sphincter to be able to suck."[28]

ANIMAL INSTINCTS

Animals play prominent and even mysterious roles in the collective stories and beyond in regards to face transplantation. Considering the fact that the students were not familiar with the details of Ms. Dinoire's situation, it is interesting to consider why animals figure so abundantly in the stories. But even beyond the collective stories animals still figure prominently in the story of facial allografts.

At some basic human level we have always struggled to distinguish ourselves from animals. Proximity to the animal kingdom is a delicate thing for most people; the closer a human gets to the world of the animal, the more likely it is for other people to dehumanize or classify that person in proximity to nature as being more animal and less human. Compelled by some fear of being near to animal nature, humans will often oscillate on a continuum from apelike to present-day human, always trying to distinguish themselves from their "animal instincts," real animals, and often from some of our fellow humans, all the while keeping a foot in the natural order of things (for instance, think of the Werner Herzog film *Grizzly Man* or the way sufferers of severe mental illness are often relegated to subhuman treatment). The precarious nature of existing on this teeter-totter of the natural world places humans in a position to feel that when the plank tips the animal kingdom and we slowly slide down from a privileged perspective to a world below, we are at risk of becoming something other than human. This is an experience that many steer clear of at all costs; an experience, however, that is—perhaps ironically—part of what it means to be a human.

Infants often serve as vivid reminders of our animal-like pasts. Babies, like animals, will defecate where and when desired, eat with fierce vigor, and lash out in anger when the urge strikes. With behaviors like these in mind, infants are often thought to exist very much in proximity with animal instincts. In the field of developmental psychological, infancy is the beginning of the long progression toward becoming ever so more human, that is, walking and talking. It is expected that we will grow out of infancy; we accept it as a stage that is to be left behind. Even in situations where humans might lapse back into infant-like behavior, such behavior is duly noted with the judgment that a person has "regressed," as, once again, sliding back down the teeter-totter of nature makes a person lose a certain sense of something that they have gained. In such a case, the loss is obvious: we have lost our humanness.

Perhaps, though, there is a different way of understanding this teeter-totter relationship with animality. What of the idea that an encounter with an animal, be it wild or domesticated, is an encounter that draws a human being out of its complacency within the "natural order" of the world, allowing them the opportunity to *gain* something of what it means to occupy a precarious position in the world with other creatures. The precarious position of finding oneself in uncharted human territory is not a precariousness that is not unique to humankind; an animal too has something to lose as well as something to gain from coming into contact with its human neighbor. No matter from which direction the encounter may be coming, the idea remains the same for both humans and animals: contact with something foreign and unfamiliar necessarily entails a transforming view of one's world. Borders change as the world one inhabits changes.

In her recent book, *When Species Meet*, noted figure in the posthumanities Donna J. Haraway outlines a way of experiencing the interrelationships shared by living things in what she calls "companion species," a descriptive way of taking up the interacting[29] creatures of the earth in a way that is not categorical, but rather, "a pointer to an ongoing 'becoming with.'"[30] Throughout her book, Haraway evokes many examples of

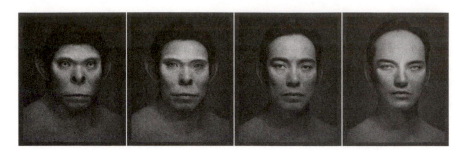

Daniel Lee, Self-Portraits, 1997. Courtesy of Daniel Lee

"companion species" or "messmates,"[31] often referencing technology, art, science, and relationships with domesticated animals with the purpose of not only advocating for a symbiotic understanding of individuals, but also challenging traditionally defined limits in which humans place various sorts of animate and inanimate entities.

What is compelling about Haraway's notion of companion species is the way it bypasses the problematic way in which humankind perceives itself in a privileged position over other entities with which it shares the world. By suggesting that "partners do not precede their relating; all that is, is the fruit of becoming with,"[32] Haraway points to a way of conceiving of the "natural world" in a movement where the teeter-totter of nature is no longer defined by vertigo, but by an ongoing, indefinite undulation that draws living creatures into an evolving process of redefining the natural world—and a human being's position within it.

FACES, PETS, AND COMPANIONS

It must be noted that two out of the four cases of face transplantation have involved animals. Dinoire, of course, lost her face while the family dog pawed at her as she lay in a drug-induced sleep. The face of the second face transplant recipient was removed by a bear as he chased it off with a stick, trying to protect his sheep herd, and the third facial allograft was on a French man who suffered from the rare genetic Von Recklinghausen's disease, otherwise called "Elephant Man's disease." Recall the infamous case of John Merrick made popular in David Lynch's film *Elephant Man*. Remarkably, and most recently, after "Travis" the Chimpanzee ripped off Charla Nash's face in Stamford, Connecticut, the victim was stabilized and the transferred to the face transplant ward at The Cleveland Clinic. Face transplantation has been mentioned in two other animal attacks, one by a pig in China on a little girl and another in the United States in a case where a two-year-old boy's face was removed by a pitbull terrier.

Face transplantation elevates us from a raw animal state back into the world of humankind. The facial allograft works to not only propel us forward ahead at the level of technology but also at the level of understanding more subtle and psychologically complex aspects of ourselves. Boundaries, the grotesque, and identity all converge with the animal aspects associated with face transplants. Pascal Coler's face having been attacked by an elephantine disease is transformed from its grotesque elephant disease animal state into a very passable human form, one that permits him to even "find a wife, settle down, and have children."[33] With these wishes he expressed the most human of human traits: companionship, love, and the desire for reproduction. The transplant has permitted him to burst out of the animalistic barrier preventing him from being fully human. The transplant liberates him from the barriers of the grotesque and provides him with a new identity where his hopes and dreams can come true. "I even dream of myself in my new face."[34]

Although it might be odd that so many references to animals crop up when talking about face transplants, the fear of somehow turning into an animal, or, clearer yet, an unidentifiable "creature," makes sense when viewed in the context of what people fear they would be losing in receiving a face transplant: the distinct quality of being a human. Somewhere in the experience of the face transplant itself, beyond the presence of any animals, lies a way of taking up Haraway's idea of companion species in relation to face transplant procedures. The recipients of the face transplant themselves have had their identity as "normal" human beings altered, becoming the image of a human being who many people are not quite able to yet catch up to. Perhaps the individual who emerges from having received a face transplant is no longer human in a traditional sense; it is possible that, as a result of a face transplant, the recipient has developed into a companion species version of good old fashioned "mankind." As such, the face transplant is an example of a sort of "becoming-with" for humans, an amorphous image of the future in which the truly precarious position of all entities that exist in the world become and remain precariously situated; the human is never quite human, nor ever quite animal.

It is this gray area of definition to which face transplants take people, as amply evidenced in the fantasies people have of face transplants, which is simply unfathomable for any person stuck on the idea of a set and fixed understanding of what a human being is. If one of the major binaries under which this vision labors is "man" vs. animal, it would seem natural that when an individual that is no longer quite "man" (but perhaps more fully "human") is encountered, that the first word that might come to mind is "animal."

Going along with Haraway's idea of the "less shapely and more rambunctious"[35] notion of the "companion species," there is something very amorphic about the experience of losing one's face and identity on the one hand and having an exchange with an animal that does not quite seem to fit into simple "man/animal" categorization. After all, Dinoire's dog, as many news reports liked to believe, was only trying to wake her up in the best Lassie-like fashion imaginable, but which, as a result of the injury that the dog created for Dinoire, was simply unfathomable for those who put the dog to sleep. With such a loss of definition as experienced in an "animal encounter," people likely feel violated, and in the case of Dinoire and her dog, exacted justice (or revenge) on Dinoire's dog for aiding her in exceeding a boundary of humanness. Part of what it means to coexist alongside other creatures is that the contact of such a shared world will inevitably result in the change and redefinition of individuals within that world. However, an understanding of shared change within the natural world among different entities is an idea that trucks very little with a world defined through the privileged position of humankind. Ultimately, the encounter with animals and all of the associations with animality that the sort of "becoming-with," to again use Haraway's phrase, that a face transplant implies concerns the overwhelming fear and anxiety that human beings encounter when they are confronted with an image of the future of humans, an image of what they could become. The specific challenge to what it means to be human that a face transplant implies is much easier to dismiss when it is viewed as somehow being "animal," that is, beneath the dignity of humans. Although the results of our narrative exercise with groups of students do not necessarily result in strict defensive denials of challenging aspects of face transplant procedures, the puzzling references to animality found in the students' responses seem to indicate something of the fears we are here addressing. It is almost as if the responses were saying that because a face transplant does not adhere to a conventional vision of what a human being is, any recipient is somehow less than or other than what any other human being is. Rather than understand this data as a retreat a conventional view of humanness, might not this data be pointing to a more extraordinary vision of what it means to be human?

FINAL ASSOCIATIONS

There are some quirks about the story results that deserve further attention. For example, why is it that topics such as surgery, blood, and knives—topics you would think are areas of high concern when dealing with this type of surgery—take up so little of the fantasy stories? If the exercise is supposed to be one of un-repression, of playfully freeing the unconscious, the results are curious. What one expects to be concerns surrounding the topic of surgery, such as blood, death, and scars, turn out not to be very prevalent as responses. It could be that these topics are highly psychically dangerous and are under repression. They are locked so deeply away that the group story-writing technique leaves them undisturbed. Another way to understand this result is to think of it in light of a spatial relationship where the highest level responses wrap back around to connect with the low-level response in a kind of Möbius strip. Here, the low level comments are a kind of underside of the most common. Perhaps residing beneath how one eats with a transplanted face is the fear of death, beneath fears that face is not stable exists the topic of scars and blood. Each anxiety has an underside, a deeper and darker, yet more repressed relative.

This sample of responses from a fairly typical American college classroom is suggestive of certain themes and responses that face transplant procedures seem to provoke. The many remarkable and often puzzling responses we see in these student responses are certainly not incidental. Far from flukes, these responses are merely representative of similar fantasies, associations, and fears that can be found at more accessible and familiar levels in popular culture such as literature and film.

THE OUTER LIMITS

With associations to stories such as Frankenstein, face transplant procedures have a certain science fiction quality. Transplants, as marvels of modern medicine, are often taken up in mythical dialogue as a way of examining their features, faults, and future. The most famous example of this kind of literary allusion to unprecedented procedures is, as we discussed in the introduction to this book, *Frankenstein*. Indeed, *Frankenstein* was, without a doubt, a story that often came to mind when people learned about the performance of the world's first successful face transplants. In what is the most accurate portrayal of a face transplant in popular culture, the French horror film *Eyes Without a Face* (1959) is the story of a face transplant cast in a terrifying light. The story of Dr. Genessier, a celebrated surgeon and his daughter, Christine, whose face was left disfigured in a car wreck caused by Dr. Genessier, *Eyes Without a Face* follows Dr. Genessier's quest to restore a beautiful visage to his daughter. The means through which the doctor pursues this goal, however, are quite different from that of today's transplant surgeons. With the aid of his assistant, Genessier kidnaps young women whose faces look similar to his daughter's, bringing them back to his institution, whereupon he anesthetizes the women and removes their faces, leaving the women for dead while he transplants their faces onto the head of his daughter. Including an extended sequence where the audience watches Genessier remove the face of a young woman, the film shows Genessier repeatedly failing to perform a successful face transplant for his daughter. Time after time Dr. Genessier's attempts at transplanting a face onto his daughter are unsuccessful, as each transplanted face fails to adhere to his daughter's head, eventually driving his daughter, wrought with sorrow over the tragic loss of her life, her boyfriend, and her face because of her disfigurement, to eventually put an end to her father's guilt driven madness. When her father had, yet again, kidnapped a young woman with the intent of stealing her face, Christine helped the woman escape from her father's institute, releasing the dogs that her father practices procedures on. After the girl escapes, the film ends with a shot of the dogs attacking Doctor Genessier, biting him on his face, a fitting and rather ironic end given the circumstances surrounding the world's first face transplant.

This film, intended as a modern remake of Frankenstein, was not only prescient in the specific ways that it built a sense of horror and fear into the face transplant experience, it was even somehow correct about the first nation that would perform the procedure—France. Beyond the startling prediction that this film seems to make about the procedure (the progress montage of Genessier's daughter's transplanted face being rejected is especially uncanny), the film seems to drive at fears attached to the procedure that we have already hinted at: loss of self, worry over being violated, and animal attacks. As a continuation of the Frankenstein myth, *Eyes Without a Face* serves as a cautionary tale over the uses of science—but it also seems to say that identity is one thing that we can never lose.

The terror of identity loss, of somehow having one's self violated, does not only manifest itself in horror films. In an episode of the immensely popular television show from the Disney Channel show *Hannah Montana,* titled "Achy Jakey Heart," Miley Cyrus's character, normal Miley Stewart by day and pop phenom Hannah Montana by night, faces a crisis in her courtship with a boy: she must decide whether or not to reveal her "true" self as Hannah Montana to her boyfriend, the famous actor Jake. As the episode moves on, Miley learns that Jake himself, as a celebrity, is really a boy named Leslie, a fact that both struggle with in their straining to have an "ordinary" relationship. Without launching further into the dissection of a teenage romance, it is worth noting that at one point during the episode, Miley, while mulling over the difficulties of her situation with Jake, tells her friend Lilly that she should either just move to Peru or get a face transplant to avoid the situation. Although the reference is not significant, it is worth noting that the reference fell in the middle of an episode where Miley is in the throws of an identity crisis, where her "true" self is at risk of being violated.

In another television show, of a decidedly more adult focus, face transplants play a central role in an episode devoted to the question of identity. "Hannah Tedesco," an episode from the FX show *Nip/Tuck*, an episode that aired a mere two weeks before Isabelle Dinoire's procedure, had its plot focused around a proposed face transplant to be performed on a young woman, Hannah Tedesco, who was disfigured on a carnival ride. Surrounding the story of the show's two main characters Christian Ford and Sean McNamara's attempt to perform the face transplant procedure, a number of subplots swell around the face transplant story line, all examining the question of identity from different vantage points: running from organized crime, entering into witness protection, and getting married. As every character seems to struggle with the question of who they are, perhaps best exemplified by a scene where Sean McNamara, while contemplating entering into witness protection with a woman he has fallen for, must burn off his fingerprints, erasing a fundamental link to his old identity in order to take start a new. However, when asked to take this bold and painful step, Sean cannot do so. Having initial success with performing the risky face transplant procedure, the show ends with Hannah Tedesco's facial allograft being rejected and the surgeons peeling off the skin from her face transplant, with all the plot lines of the episode, in some sense, back at where the episode began.

As with *Eyes Without a Face*, the facial allograft in this episode of *Nip/Tuck* doesn't simply fail to take because of an immunosuppressive problem; when viewed in the larger context of the stories to which it is attached, the procedure fails for more much more complex plot reasons: plot reasons that amount to a psychological/cultural rejection of the idea of a face transplant—much like that of the case of the Chinese man and his transplanted penis. In both *Nip/Tuck* and *Eyes Without a Face*, there is something that keeps the transplant procedures from being successes, but what is it?

IDENTITY THEFT

Delmer Daves' classic film noir *Dark Passage* (based on the David Goodis novel *Dark Street*), starring Humphrey Bogart and Lauren Bacall, takes up the theme of a layer of identity that one cannot shed in the story of a convicted criminal, Vincent Parry, on the lam from the law. Parry, a man wrongfully serving a life sentence in San Quentin for the murder of his wife, a crime he did not commit, escapes from jail, determined to find the person who did kill his wife and send him up river to be punished for the crime. In the story, Parry's character, a recognizable man, finds his way to a plastic surgeon who goes to work on Parry's face, changing his appearance altogether. The film, the first half of which is shot from a subjective angle, as to conceal the appearance of the main character, then follows Parry's attempt to redeem himself, unable to simply flee San Francisco until he locates the person responsible for his wife's murder. Bogart's character, no matter how much his appearance had changed, can't hide from the law forever and eventually has to go on the run. As Parry learns that to clear his name he must pass through the dark streets of his past, he slowly pieces together who killed his wife, but only enough to clear his name for himself, for the killer perishes before Parry ever has the chance to clear his name with the law. And yet, in spite of this circumstance in the film, we witness a Parry at the end of the film, on the coast of Mexico with Bacall in his arms, seemingly unshackled from his past; it was only ever to himself that Parry had anything to prove.

Sometimes it is not enough to change one's appearance to change one's identity, though it can certainly help. Parry wouldn't have been able to make a new attempt at life if he hadn't first donned a new face. But change can certainly hurt as well. As we find in the Japanese auteur Hiroshi Teshigahara's film adaptation of the Kobo Abe novel, *The Face of Another*, sometimes changing our appearance can only lead us further away from a traumatic past that binds us to an indefinite pain of the future. *The Face of Another* follows the tale of Okuyama, a businessman who was badly disfigured in a chemical accident, and after experiencing an immense amount of psychological pain as a result of being alienated from his wife, his friends, and his life, consults with a doctor who offers a miracle cure for Okuyama's problem: a face transplant. Developing alongside the story of a woman whose face was disfigured in the American attacks on Nagasaki in 1945, Okuyama slowly begins to become a new person, acting the part of the transplanted mask that the doctor had created for him, aiming to seduce his now alienated wife in an act of revenge. But as Okuyama begins to live a new life in accord with his new face, his life begins to spiral out of control as the distance he feels between his self and the mask grow stronger and stronger. As we find in *Dark Passage*, Okuyama's attempt to exorcise his past by effacing his appearance is not enough to overcome his ghostly past. As the victim of Nagasaki serves as a reminder throughout the film, any move forward that does not consider the scar of the past as an opportunity for transformation will only be hindered by the blindness with which it treats the past.

In the recent Bruce Wagner novel, *Memorial*, there is a bit of hyperactive dialogue among characters that, interestingly enough, is about face transplant procedures: "I mean, do you think the paranoid American doctors would try to sew a woman's face back on? That woman in France whose face got torn off by a dog? And now, she's a *fox*. Demetrius and I *love* her. She still *smokes her Gauloises*! How French is *that*. I'm telling you, that cadaver donor was a *hottie*! The Americans would be so terrified! Of being sued! But it's not their fault, it's the *system's*."[36] Written in Wagner's signature gossip-cum-poetry, Wagner not only seems to encapsulate all of the associations in a brilliant free association about face transplants, the novel from which this quote comes is an incisive examination of the very sort of problem of an identity's past that we find in *The Face of Another* and *Dark Passage*. Wagner's novel, however, probes much more deeply into the problems of a culture obsessed with feeling like a victim, a society compulsively driven to identify with traumatic experiences. The need to identify oneself as a victim, to identity with victims, and to be seen as traumatized appears as a peculiar concern in the world today. Certainly, there is an obvious link that exists between tragedy and celebrity in our culture, wherein one's failures and falls are just as definitive in the ascent of one's public identity as one's positive attributes, and although one can rationalize the link between celebrity and tragedy, it is odd that pain is something people so actively seek out. Unlike the stories of *Dark Passage* and *The Face of Another*, two stories about transforming one's past, trauma culture and the need to identify oneself as a victim use the past not as a springboard, but as a resting home. Popular culture representations of face transplants often contain these very reflections of victimhood in their plots, associations that often seek to undermine the proliferation of these procedures through fear tactics.

For instance, take the John Woo film *Face/Off*, starring John Travolta and Nicolas Cage. The film, the tale of a sting operation gone bad, concerns an archetypal bad guy-as-terrorist, initially played by Nicolas Cage, pitted against the archetypal hero-as-FBI agent initially played by John Travolta. In order to acquire the details of a bombing planned by Nicolas Cage's character, Travolta's character undergoes a face-swap with Cage's comatose character, with Travolta's character then going to the same prison as Cage's character's brother in order to get the information on the bombing plot. The plan backfires, though, when Travolta's face as Nicolas Cage's character wakes up, realizes what has occurred, and does away with the surgical staff that performed the procedure. Nicolas Cage's character then proceeds to take over the life of the FBI agent, entering into his household, sleeping with his wife, and using his job for his own criminal interests. As these sorts of stories tend to go, the bad guy gets it in the end, but not before he has the chance to try to ruin Travolta's character's face in an attempt to rob him of ever being able to return to the life he once had as an FBI agent. Aside from standard worries about the loss of one's world with the loss of one's identity, it is interesting to see the way that one's identity, and by extension one's life, depends so much on one's face. When that face is put at risk, when one stands to lose their identity, the only way of saving face, it would seem, within our culture is to become a victim, to avoid the difficulty of having one's world thoroughly disrupted.

A collective fear of experiencing some sort of identity theft, a fear that places masses of people in the position of victim, is merely a way of collectively not facing up to the challenge of having to rearticulate different levels of identity within a culture. The way we have always understood identity has come into doubt, We do not have the means to overcome the past, the accumulation of one's identity being pushed forward in time in a new articulation, in the form of a new face. Our culture's fascination with trauma and victimization, from the obsessive coverage of "Amber alerts," to 9/11 culture, reality TV shows like *Survivor*, and disaster films of varying stripes, demonstrates that the need to identify oneself as a victim is indeed a strange impulse. Some of the associations that spring forth from the films addressed above, such as *Eyes Without a Face* and *Face/Off,* present face transplant procedures in this very light of victimization, almost as if one way to deal with the shock of the procedure is to identify some person being wronged by its implementation. By casting a victim somewhere along the way in the story of a face transplant, a fear of technology not only creates the moral ground from which people can deny the dissemination of the procedure, a sanctuary identity is constructed in which people may hide from the light that face transplant procedures cast on identity and how these procedures somehow ask us to no longer victimize ourselves. The haven of victimhood is indeed a means to evade having to assess the practical, cultural, and ethical implications of face transplant procedures, allowing us to forever seek refuge in the past, in what we know, and to fear the moment where, as Sean McNamara faced in *Nip/Tuck*, we must make the decision as to whether or not we are willing to let go of certain aspects of ourselves. Although some parts of an identity cannot be willed away, to continue moving in life one must relinquish the parts of one's self that only serve to harm and stifle movement.

FACING FANTASY

There are many more references to face transplant procedures, as well as facial cosmetic surgery, that crop up throughout popular culture. Comedic references to plastic surgery one finds on a Web site such as Perezhilton. com[37] and photos and outrageous stories about Dinoire appearing in countless tabloids,[38] as well as cheap humor sites.[39] References to face transplants abound in art films, as well as gossip pages. All references to face transplant procedures invariably circulate around questions of identity. Often the examples represent story lines dealing with the procedure through the lens of many of the same fears and anxieties that are commonly attached to face transplant procedures, for example, violation of boundaries, animal encounters, loss of self, and a traumatic past one wants to overcome, as well as some aspect of a self that people seem unable to shed. Possibly the fantasies serve to support a cultural climate warm to the practice of face transplantation. Certainly the abundant representations of swapping faces with another indicate a cultural obsession at the level of identity. Before the actual facial allotransplantation these fantasies existed. No one really knows what impact the actual surgery may mean, all we can know is that face transplantation and identity deserve attention and analysis.

In the next chapter, analysis is exactly what we get. Psychoanalytic perspectives on face transplants help to uncover and digest some of these deeply seated anxieties and needs surrounding faces. Chapter 3 exposes the fantasies and provides analysis of them at the cultural level, and in Chapter 4, we turn the lens of analysis further inside and take a developmental and clinical approach. Faces, narcissism, skin envelopes, mirrors, and temporality take the center stage as face transplantation heads to the couch.

Analyzing the Face: Part I

I'M THE LOVE OF MY LIFE

In 1979, Christopher Lasch published his book *The Culture of Narcissism*. In it he presented a prescient vision of what he feared: people increasingly turning toward themselves in a selfish, self-serving, and narcissistic fashion. "To live for the moment is the prevailing passion—to live for yourself, not for your predecessors or posterity."[1] The book was a nationwide bestseller, and Lasch made some rather unnerving conclusions that hold true today. He argued that our turn toward narcissism is in part due to increasing capital wealth. We work outside of the home and turn toward "experts" to train and teach our children, instead of the preindustrial custom of teaching our own children the skills they will need to lead productive lives. We have become drivers of minivans sporting bumper stickers that read "Mom's Taxi," while children are driven around to various kinds of lessons, sports activities, playdates, and tutoring sessions. We now buy what we used to provide for free in our homes. Under our own roofs we could shape our children's tastes, talents, and skills necessary for survival, demonstrating to our children that we indeed have skills, that we are indeed competent and learned adults. It is now commonplace to purchase skills from expert others. We have become resolute that there is little to offer our children and families beyond the very basic mechanics behind child maintenance. Even the physical exercise we may be quite skilled at, swimming or jogging for example, is performed outside the view of our children in a gym or sports club. Although it effectively works against the farming out of children to others for training and skills for academic learning, the homeschooling movement still does not reverse the trend completely. Most homeschooled children share a curriculum purchased online. Therefore, homeschooling does not really demonstrate a reversal of the trend. The knowledge in the textbooks and computer programs is not generated from the parents themselves.

Lasch makes cutting points regarding the dangers of not teaching children in the home what we know and how to excel. Without instruction the home becomes what he describes in another of his books, *Haven in a Heartless World: The Family Besieged.*"[2] Here, the home devoid of economic, scholarly, and trade functions serves only to comfort and coddle. Parents hide their expertise and the quality of their working mind. Lasch argues in the *Haven* book that family life has been rendered down to the parental duties of making sure children feel safe and secure. Note how many children's catalogs feature safety gates, safety latches, and boo-boo bunnies. Parents turn to books on how to raise their infants and children as if their sole investment and gift to their offspring are child-raising techniques as prescribed by others. The parent advice book *What to Expect When You're Expecting* has been on *The New York Times* bestseller list for more than 350 weeks.[3] Oddly, when comparing one parenting book to another, it is revealed that they are almost universally in conflict with one another. Take breast-feeding for instance; information on how to do it is wildly divergent depending on whom one reads. Feed on demand any time of day, put the baby on a schedule, empty one breast then switch, feed five minutes on one and switch baby over, let baby fall asleep at the breast, make sure they fall asleep off the breast, and so on. The take-home message of all this confusing advice may be that there is no right or wrong way. Infants will demand food, and it will be given one way or another. The advice really just stands alone as advice, something to be turned to when fears of inadequacy arise when one brings the baby home and it cries and must be fed. The key point is that the impulse is indeed to reach outside of oneself toward a bookshelf: bibliotherapy.

Even with a critical awareness it is practically impossible to avoid reading at least some parenting literature and not taking it seriously because the business of taking care of little children is stressful, demanding, and challenging at so many levels. However, it seems that family chaos is not dealt with strategically or effectively, increasing confusion and augmenting parental concerns that they cannot be their own experts. Certainly more pieces of compelling evidence of our feeling adrift in our own homes can be found in the myriad of reality-based television programs, such as *Dr. Phil,* that try to amend broken families. Other popular shows, such as

Jon & Kate Plus Ei8ht, aim to display family chaos. Jon and Kate cope with their young twin daughters and a younger set of sextuplets. Family pathology takes center stage just for the sake of savage amusement on other television programs. The "Octo Mom," who gave birth to eight newborns, promises much more of the same.

Nanny-based shows are popular on television. This genre of programming best highlights family problems and the expert advice to fix them—on the spot via home-based assistance. These television shows, if anything, speak to an increasing and chronic need to find direction through the parenting maze. Even if viewed as a form of entertainment, the pleasures derived from a show like *Nanny 911* come in the form of watching the pack of wild and untamed kids push their bumbling and bewildered parents to the brink of insanity. Then, viola, arriving in the back of a chaffered London taxicab enters nanny sporting a natty woolen cap and caped uniform. Unlike the parents she comes to train and the children she comes to tame, she is singularity unflappable and always, repeat always, successful. There is a deeply embedded kind of colonist fantasy at work here. Like strangers in a new land, yet still oddly within our own homes, we flounder about trying to tame the natives who seem so much more in control and savvy about the ways of the new world. With a bit of admitted chagrin a call is sent out for the rescue troops. With time, like ships sailing across the Atlantic, cruise ashore the nanny squadrons. Who else other than the British, arguably the world's most accomplished colonists, could help us to better master and civilize the little monkeys that live in our midst?

The admission of needing help is one thing, but this is clearly not the case being played out in the nanny scenario. Rather, what is displayed is Lasch's observation that confidence is garnered only through the approval of outside experts. The ultimate price paid is when our own healthy self-love and narcissism become possible only through the approving nods and back pats of others. The requirement that sources outside of our own creation are needed to provide ourselves feelings of well-being, combined with the assumed need that by purchasing products, skills, services, and advice we will succeed, ironically heightens a form of unhealthy narcissism. Here Lasch explains how:

> Narcissism represents the psychological dimension of this dependence. Notwithstanding his occasional illusions of omnipotence, the narcissist depends on others to validate his self-esteem. He cannot live without an admiring audience. His apparent freedom from family ties and institutional constraints does not free him to stand alone or to glory his individuality. On the contrary, it contributes to his insecurity, which he can overcome only by seeing his "grandiose self" reflected in the attentions of others, or by attaching himself to those who radiate celebrity, power, and charisma.[4]

As a practical application and explanation of the Lasch quote, we can return to the disenfranchised parent. Finding themselves caught alone among the savages within the home, mommy and daddy need supernanny's assistance, and ultimately supernanny's super approval, to gain feelings of personal worth and self-love. Adults in this scenario live for the attentions of others with dire needs to be admired by others in a kind of starvation for self-love. The world becomes our mirror and we scan it for signs of our worthiness.

In the TLC television hit *What Not to Wear*, the mirror once again plays a role in dispensing a shiny and admiring reflection, this time on the fashion illiterate. In this program, friends and family nominate coworkers or sisters who simply cannot chose the correct wardrobe and require expert advice. The show's wardrobe savants and cohosts Stacy and Clinton are called to the rescue. After the ritual ceremonial closet invasion, a barrage of humiliating comments, and trashing of the lucky nominee's entire wardrobe, she is given a large sum of money to purchase new clothes. However, she must adhere to the advice of the duo's strict dos and don'ts of purchasing.

Although the show can be celebrated for the positive self-esteem message, the message is ultimately about the culling of beauty through the guidance and approval of a team of experts. The fashion professionals can guide any hausfrau toward a look guaranteed to make her neighbors and coworkers jump in delight during the final reveal. Equally as unflappable as supernanny standing in a whirlwind of out-of-control children, the beauty experts in *What Not to Wear* never pooh-pooh a single body type or stringy hairdo. Even the most drab hair or blotchy skin has a glowing potential that can be unleashed by the show's hair and makeup wizards. The final scenes of every episode are pure Lasch-like fodder. The once-frumpy gal parades her coifed and radiant self out toward a full-length mirror where Clinton and Stacy await. After an extended session of the approving cohost's sly winks to one another, the show concludes with the contestant going home. Once in her hometown she is greeted by her waiting and usually thrilled family and friends who surround and applaud the new and improved version before their eyes. We have become a culture of externally generated narcissists indeed. Ability to soothe ourselves and repair our own egos has been damaged in these narcissistic times.

THE PSYCHODYNAMICS OF NARCISSISM

Importantly, it is from within this culture of narcissism that springs the implementation of external body allotransplantations like hands and faces. Perhaps it is only within a societal structure driven by narcissistic forces that face transplantations actually become more than fantasy. Clearly film and television have toyed with the idea for a long time, but to actually perform the operative procedure requires a strong supportive cultural interest to "just do it." By looking through the lens of a psychoanalytic theory sensitive to narcissistic human elements, one can scrape away some of the layers underneath the conscious surface of how face transplantation might work, that is, what is the "it" of "just do it." Ultimately, the goal is to shed light on a still unexplored aspect of emergent technology.

To explore anxieties about both narcissism and face transplantation two psychodynamic theorists from the object relations school are discussed. Through the object relations lens it is possible to glean understanding of the relationship between how we initially learn to become a nonpart of another human being. Object relations theory also provides a way to more deeply understand the psychological dynamics inherent in narcissism. The theory also permits a fresh approach to thinking about face transplantations, both for a potential face allograft recipient and as a reactionary audience.

Specifically, the two psychoanalytic theorists used here are both English object relations theorists: Melanie Klein and Donald Winnicott. Klein was a child psychoanalyst who believed that Freud's theory left too much unsaid about the very earliest of human years. Object relations theory proposes that the human psyche is well developed by the age of two. Klein's three-stage developmental theory, in fact, completely unfolds during the first couple years of life. Her theory is an excellent introduction to object relations theory because of the very vivid and accessible way it can be described. To the uninitiated, the word "object" may seem an awkward way to discuss human relationships. However, if one considers the world from the infant's point of view, there are only objects at first: no relationships, no fathers or mothers, only objects that mysteriously come and go. For Klein, the infant's world is split into objects that bring pleasure and relief from hunger and objects that appear to deliver the pains of hunger and other negative bodily sensations. The tiny infant has no way to know that the discomfort of hunger or the pressure of gas is caused by its own body. All the baby knows is that some objects deliver great comfort and some objects deliver very bad treatment. Klein calls this splitting of the world into all good and all bad the baby's first coping mechanism. By splitting the world into these simple terms the infant can draw in as much of the good it can take by greedily sucking milk and absorbing all comforting touches. Likewise, Klein hypothesized that the infant will fantasize defending itself from the terrible ravages it feels are attacking and destroying its feelings of well-being. After all, if good comes from the outside, then most certainly these aggravations and pains must too be from the outside.[5]

Hollywood has taken these very primitive fears that we have all shared in infancy and used them to generate some of the more terrifying science fiction films to date. A classic Kleinian type of story line is the film *Aliens,* where bad objects get inside bodies and cause terror and ultimately death.[6] Recall the scene where the Sigourney Weaver character lies on the table and a small object travels beneath her skin until it bursts out. The film *The Matrix* uses a similar scene.[7] For an object relations theorist it is this kind of scene where something very bad from the outside gets inside, threatening annihilation, which unnerves us to our very core. We dread at an unconscious level what we lived as an infant baby. For better or worse, Klein refers to this splitting in terms of the giving "good breast" and persecutory "bad breast." This concept has even been adopted in a Hollywood film. Woody Allen, notorious for his long personal history with psychoanalytic treatment, used an amusing scene in his 1972 film *Everything You Ever Wanted to Know About Sex* But Were Afraid to Ask.*[8] In one segment, Allen films a mock-up of a gigantic breast that kills everything is its path by squirting milk out a huge nipple. One of the better gag lines is when Allen kneels next to one of the victims and says, "The milk slowed him down, but it was the cream that killed him." Allen brings to the big screen a humorous take on Klein's theory of the bad persecutory breast.

For Klein it is a developmental necessity that we move out of this world of splitting and enter what she called the depressive position. Here the baby at around six months of age begins to realize that the good object and the bad object are actually connected to the same one object, that of its caretaker. Thus a crisis develops around this tension, and the infant must reconcile the fact that it has been fantasizing about defending itself and attacking the good object and the bad object at the same time. Klein calls this stage the depressive position. When one thinks of baby's tears at this half-year age, they are often attributed it to the pain of teething. Perhaps this is true, but Klein makes us also consider that crying at this stage can also signal a psychic unease that emerges out of the realization that mommy is both a good and bad object. Anxiety arises out of a dawning awareness that they have invested energy in trying to harm her. The way out of this dilemma is to find relief through acts of reparation, Klein's last stage. How better to soothe the fears that we have damaged another's well-being other than making up for it and bringing healing. Thus toddlers spend a lot of their time patting adult's backs when they think they seem sad, pushing morsels of food into their mouths, and walking about the house finding little treasures to deliver into the welcoming hands of a grownup. Yes, some adults are more or less arrested at the splitting stage and lump all their experiences into either very good or very bad. Yes, some adults live in anxious and fearful psychic worlds where they feel guilty and afraid their whole lives, and, of course, some adults have not developed abilities to make up after real or imagined transgressions and heal the ones they love.

A FACE IN THE MIRROR

English child psychoanalyst Donald Winnicott famously wrote, "in individual emotional development *the precursor of the mirror is the mother's face.*"[9] He posited that one can understand an adult's emotional life through examination of their mirror relations. How we experience our own face and understand the facial communication of others is central to Winnicott's ideas about what constitutes mental health. Social interaction for little babies consists primarily of face gazing. According to Winnicott, adult faces serve as mirroring, reflective surfaces. The role of the adult face is not to present a version of their own face to the baby, but rather, to mimic the baby's expression. Winnicott's theory begins with the tiny infant's gaze out into the landscape, scanning the faces of the environment. There they encounter a kind of reflective surface where their own face can be mirrored back. Psychologically healthy adults will naturally do this act of mirroring—that is, being capable of temporarily relinquishing their own internal world in order to reflect back the baby's own face. Think about how one naturally does this "looking back" when holding a baby. The baby hiccups and one usually hiccups back; the baby smiles, and one smiles back. Maybe the mirroring occurs in an exaggerated sense, but the baby typically takes the lead, and the adult gives back not the exact same face, but a proximally close imitation. Most importantly, the baby learns what their reflection is like in the face of another. It is from this mirroring psychodynamic relationship that one develops two crucial emotionally healthy ways of being.

First, the baby learns that their spontaneous expressions, whether they are happy or sad, playful, or serious, are regarded as such and are accepted as such in an uncritical and unfettered fashion. If accomplished, this sense of "real me" can emerge over the course of babyhood. Second, and just as importantly, the baby begins to learn how to see itself through the face of another. In a metaphorical sense, a me-not-me slowly emerges. In essence, the baby says to itself, "when I look in that face, I see somebody who feels familiar to me, I think it is me, but it's a kind of creative seeing of me, a kind of facial poetics." Indeed, learning to look into a mirror as poetry, to see oneself as a mélange of myself as part feeling, part seeing, pure spontaneity, and part interpretation of me is essential to healthy emotional growth. Winnicott called this way of seeing *apperception.*

As a case illustration and further explanation of how faces matter to emotional development, Winnicott speaks of the self-portraits of painter Francis Bacon. Bacon's self-portraits have what Winnicott called a maddening twist: "seeing himself in his mother's face, but with some twist in him or her that maddens both him and us."[10] At first read, Bacon's face paintings would seem to signal pathology and emotional disruption—the way *not* to proceed. However, far from being completely negative, even if this twist indeed reflects a distorted and maybe even somewhat pathological externalization of his internal world, it is ultimately a creative way of portraying one's face. For Winnicott, to comprehend one's face as a creative act is necessary to avoid the traps of seeing the face too literally. Bacon is seeing his face with imagination, a metaphor or perhaps even a poem of his reflection. He is using apperception. Furthermore, one who can use apperception with themselves can also use it to look at the face of others. That is, to see the face of a friend or lover as more than just surface beauty. Apperceivers are attracted to what is under the skin because they already know how to delve beneath their own.

The alternative to creative mirror gazing is literal mirror gazing, that is, looking in the mirror and seeing a real face, with real pores, real acne, real wrinkles; Winnicott refers to this noncreative kind of looking as *perception*. Consider the effects of caregiver faces that chronically offer the infant, not the opportunity to see itself, but the face of the mother who "reflects her own mood or, worse still, the rigidity of her own defenses."[11] This rigidity can have many sources. Perhaps the infant received a consistent depressive face from the caregiver whereby they presented their own emotional surface to the infant as a nonreflective surface. In a laboratory setting developmental psychologist Ed Tronick tested what would happen if mothers were asked to stop reflecting their baby's faces and instead made a neutral face.[12] He demonstrated that babies would try and engage the mother and would gradually look away and become disengaged and upset and acquire a kind of depressive face—all within a matter of minutes. In these experimental settings the effects are short lived. In Winnicott's theory of perception, infants scan the surface of the face and understand themselves and others. A "mirror is a thing to be looked at but not to be looked into."[13]

Ultimately a repetition of perceptive seeing leads to the warping of the baby's expression of spontaneous impulse. Another's face becomes one to look at, an object to be forecast like weather, not to be apperceived, but to be perceived. Learning only how to perceive, for Winnicott, places the baby and later the child and adult, into a world of perpetual emptiness. Long accustomed to reading the faces of others for clues on how they should feel, their capacity to access their inner world has significantly withered away. The adult experiences this inner world as false, and they feel empty and out of touch with how they experience the world; Winnicott called this state the "false self." Sadly, seeing this actual face of oneself can only lead to shallow self and other love. They possess little idea of how to delve and effectively relate emotionally under their own, or another's, surface.

Consider, for example, a face like entertainer Michael Jackson. Although one can only speculate on why he changes his facial features, it is interesting how many changes his face has undergone. Although he claims that his looks have only been altered because of "aging," there does seem to be a kind of obsession he has with his visage, and it makes one wonder if he sees a real face in the mirror. Does the "man in the mirror" haunt him because he sees his actual face, and not a kind of Baconian metaphorical reflection? Imagine holding a hand mirror up to your face, what might you say *you* see?

There is a passage in Lucy Grealy's book *Autobiography of a Face*—a story that chronicles her history of suffering as a child with cancer of the jaw— where she looks in the mirror. In this part of the book, Lucy reports feeling like she is seeing her literal face for the first time. Lucy had just spent the day with her mother to be fitted for an expensive wig made of real human hair. Ultimately, even after the shopkeeper and her mother convincingly tell her that the hair piece makes her beautiful, she rejects it as "ugly and awful." Yet, later that night, she becomes intrigued thinking about the shop owner's kind comments. While gazing, she keeps thinking about how he had said that she had looked terrific while trying on his hair pieces:

> I turned on the lights and very carefully assessed my face in the mirror. I was bald, but I knew that already. I also knew I had buck teeth, something I was vaguely ashamed of but hadn't given too much thought to until this moment. My teeth were ugly. And, I noticed, they were made worse by the fact that my chin seemed so small. How had it gotten that way? I didn't remember it being that small before. I rooted around in the cabinets and came up with a hand mirror and, with a bit of angling, looked for the first time at my right profile. I knew to expect a scar, but how had my face sunk in like that? I didn't understand. Was it possible I'd looked this way for a while and was only just noticing it, or was this change very recent?[14]

Her face, disfigured by her disease, turns Lucy into a Winnicottian perceiver of herself. One can only presume that she had apperceived her face before this experience and something about the wig maker event opened up awareness of her real physical status. It is hard to say whether her experience of having a facial distortion is similar to other disfigured individuals. Considering

Winnicott's theory, any traumatic facial injury would awaken both perception, such as the necessity to reconcile the injury itself, and apperception. That is, in order to go on living with one's new face a creative looking coping mechanism has to occur. Face transplantation, in light of Winnicott's theory is a newly realized and highly dynamic way to see creatively. Isabelle Dinoire's comments about her experience open an innovative door into even more ways of "seeing" than ever imagined by Winnicott himself.

WHOSE FACE IN THE MIRROR?

Isabelle Dinoire has been quoted as saying that she can only understand her new look as a form of aging, that is, that her changed appearance is due to having gotten older. Oddly, the partial face transplant does indeed create a kind of aging effect. The stitched-on face creates lines along the cheek pads that mimic the natural effects of aging. Nevertheless, imagine attempting to engage with a mirror when the face you are wearing is not your own. The face reflected back to you since the beginning of life is gone. Even the disfigured face you once had could be identified as your own—disfigured or not. But now, with the reality of face transplantation, you can wear the face of another. Gone is your own face, and it is replaced by a stranger's. What kinds of Winnicottian facial dynamics might transpire? If Dinoire's comment is examined in light of the theories of apperception and perception, it is possible to begin to divine the effect of a face transplant patient's mirror experience. Although Isabelle has commented that she feels her face is indeed now hers and that she has gotten used to it, she has also stated that every time she looks at her face in the mirror, she thinks of the donor. She has had strange alienating experiences with her face and once commented to a family member that her nose was itchy and then retracted the comment and replaced it with, "that's nonsense. It's not my nose. I have a nose that is itching."[15] She has expressed surprise that she has some facial hair on her chin that she did not have before the surgery.[16] This complaint, considering the extent of facial change that she has undergone, does indeed seem rather blasé. However, the comment does speak to profound identity-related issues. She hints that perhaps she quite frequently brings to consciousness that she is not wearing her own face.

If one's self-awareness emerges though the face one is born with, would it matter if the face is not just radically altered by plastic surgery, or injury, but replaced with the face of another? Apperception is initiated through the gift of another's ability to give themselves back to you through their interpretative mirroring of your face. Therefore, by wearing the face of another, you become simultaneously both the giver and the receiver. To wear the face of another and to make it conform to your emotions and internal life, one serves as both being a mirror for oneself—by virtue that one would now wear the other's face—and also maintaining the role of spontaneous player. This is a most perplexing psychological position. One must now perceive the face of another who is actually reflecting the perfect mirror back, but the face of the other is now the literal face of oneself—both an enviable position, in that one could always find the perfect reflection of another, but also the most potentially psychologically devastating position. Now one must confront the reality that the perfect reflection is a composite of your own face and another's. The face transplant patient is in the unique position of reading the face of another when looking in the mirror. The face may provide apperception or perception, depending on how the reflection is psychically experienced. From this object relational standpoint, wearing the face of another is to become completely alone: the most severe form of Winnicottian terror. Face transplant technology has opened doors for further exploration of narcissism and also offers new ways to understand the complexities of faces, what they mean to us psychologically and the impact of both our own and other's sense of self.

BUILDING WALL-Es

Another primary psychological warping of culture today is the lack of boundaries that are often exhibited in testing personal and technological limits. Perhaps only in this culture could the notion that the usual boundary between self and other could be so easily transgressed and that the very idea of a transplanted face would emerge without much attention outside the medical literature or even within the general population. The summer 2007 press release by Boston's Brigham and Women's Hospital stated that they may be the location of the next facial allotransplantation. This pronouncement was met without any discernable public or medical resistance or debate. Perhaps this apparent disinterest is an indicator of something a bit more concerning. Perhaps boundaries, even those as apparent as one's face as being different from another's, have begun to blur. Perhaps our identities as separate individuals from one another have begun to blur also. A powerful way to explore this question is to examine cultural trends for evidence of boundary violations and confusion.

In the summer blockbuster film *WALL-E,* a little robot routinely replaces parts of his self scavenged from the other broken robots strewn about in the film's deserted landscape of postindustrial waste.[17] There is one scene toward the end of the film where he is reconstructed almost in his entirety with replacement parts after a series of violent encounters. Once piecemealed back together, there is a long moment where he is obviously functional again, but we are unsure if he will still be himself. After a suspenseful pause, his characteristic mannerisms slowly appear, and it is clear that he indeed he does have the same personality that we grew to know previous to the extensive transplantations.

Although it may seem inane to use a children's film to make such an important point, the film highlights a contemporary concern with the concept of identity and body interchangeability. In fact, the film pulls together two cultural concerns: that of the feasibility and consequences of transplantations, and the green movement, which can be argued to be a variation of the theme of boundaries. Linked by their shared emphasis on reduce, reuse, and recycling, transplantation and environmental concerns merge together by asking similar questions about what is what and who is who after one has transferred one substance and made it into another. A soft fleece vest is made out of recycled plastic soda bottles: so what is it exactly, soft cloth or a fluffy piece of plastic? Technological advances have enabled the morphing of one object deftly into another and questions will arise, even at an unconscious level, about what exactly the recycled object is that one is holding. Body transplantations have a similar amorphous quality. How much of one human can we transplant onto another before it becomes the other person more than the recipient.

Much of the face transplant material works at this level. In fact, doing a partial face transplantation was supposed to eliminate much of the debate of what the recipient would look like versus a full face transplant, whereby the entire forehead on down to the neck is placed on another's face. It is noteworthy that the face of Pascal Coler, the third transplant recipient was, compared to the other two recipients, the closest to what is considered a full face transplant. Because his face was in excess of the typical face, that is, completely covered with huge tumors and skin boils, his facial identity was unknown from the start; that is, his real face had always been somewhat concealed. Replacing his face with someone else's gave him a face he'd never had, no firm healthy facial identity had ever been established, and nobody can even assess if he looks more like the donor or his "old" self, because he never really had a chance to have a normal face. The triangle patch would put off the worries of becoming too much like the donor, but in a culture awash with anxiety over melting polar ice caps, towering landfills, and polluted oceans, topics such as face transplantation seem to arise and become quickly adopted in the already established dialogues of the necessity of reusing and the necessity of accepting that one's own refuse will remerge in another form, blended and erased of one form and emerging as another. Like the theme of *WALL-E*, we have come to believe that it is, at least in part, life saving—both for the planet and for our bodies—to lose our boundaries.

Maybe only in a culture awash in boundary issues would there be a general lack of interest in what types of boundary transgressions, identity issues, and so on occur at an unconscious level when a person's hand, penis, or face is removed and placed on another human. But can this cultural second natured-ness of external body transplants also be a sign of something a bit more worrisome? In other words, what would it imply about mental wellness if something as inherently as unusual and conceptually amazing as face transplantation does not receive extensive examination? Perhaps it is not the case that the topic of facial allografts have been collapsed into "green" dialogs and perhaps it is not the case that we are so awash in boundary issues that the topic is viewed as offhand—especially because the topic of face transplantation often leads to an immense amount of interest even in the most casual of conversations. Rather, face transplants are difficult to talk about at some level because they unearth some of the most fundamental fears that we have about ourselves. In fact they may do this more effectively than other boundary-erasing topics, such as recycling. Psychoanalytic theory suggests that underneath us all exists the primal fear that we are not separate beings but instead beings always teetering on the edge of ourselves and with the involuntary merging with another, with the resultant fearful loss of our own sense of self. It very well may be that face transplantation represents the ultimate human desire to merge as one with another and the ultimate human fear that we might merge and lose our identity and disappear altogether.

As further evidence that boundary issues are a prevalent cultural concern, consider the most common forms of mental illnesses. Personality disabilities such as borderline personality disorder and eating disorders share a common concern with boundaries and boundary transgressions. They also share the distinction of being some of the most common forms of mental distress today. Furthermore, while only a small portion of the general population is diagnosable with an eating disorder, it can be said that on a broader spectrum we are each somewhat eating disordered, narcissistic, and borderline—that we all suffer at some level on the spectrum from these maladies. Explaining how we arrived at that point, if this is the case, is difficult to trace. Obviously there are many factors—gender related (issues related to style and appropriate behaviors), economic (issues related to poverty and family stress), global (wars and boundary tension), individual (genetics and personality), and social (expectations for contact with others). The exact cocktail recipe itself may have to remain a mystery; however, there is ample evidence to suggest that we are indeed an eating-disordered, narcissistic, and borderline culture.

While eating disorders may not be our first association to face transplantations, they have to do with testing the limits of one's own skin. Perhaps more than a gaining or losing of weight, binging and starvation are measured through changes related to one's relationship to skin. The binger or compulsive overeater wonders how far their skin will stretch. The film *Supersize Me* plays on this theme of stretching by adherence to a diet of McDonald's food.[18] The anorexic in the mirror studies not weight loss per se, but rather the relationship between the mirror image and the look of the bone-containing skin, a fact so obvious, it has almost become cliché to talk about our cultural focus on food. Whether it be dieting, fast food, portion distortion, Iron Chef, and so on, by adopting a focus on skin manipulation as the basis of these food related topics, a fresh perspective on attitudes emerges for understanding face transplantation.

AN EGO BOUNDARY OF SKIN

Unlike object relations theorists, ego psychologists are more concerned with developmental issues of consciousness and the formation of the more reality-based aspects of the self, such as the ego. It is the ego's job to regulate the primitive impulses of the id and to deal with the harsh demands of the superego. Sitting in the middle like a judge, the ego belongs to rationality and reason and balances all the incoming information it receives, protecting itself with defense mechanisms. In 1936, Sigmund Freud's youngest daughter Anna Freud published perhaps the most important early book on defense mechanisms. In it she explains the many different ways that we each learn how to protect our egos from feeling trampled by the daily harshness of social interactions.[19] If one is looked at in a way that feels belittling, or if we are prevented from realizing our goals, then the ego provides a protection whereby we defend ourselves from feeling devalued. One may, for example, have a temper tantrum and doing so regress to an earlier emotional life stage to ward off feelings of inadequacy. Or, one may redirect the feelings of aggression toward an oppressive boss and displace them onto those living at home with you. Far from being a complete negative, defense mechanisms act like quick emotional fixes. They are fast temporary ego Band-Aids to get us through our day-to-day existence. Certainly we are neurotic when we use them, but, as Freud taught us, the best you get to be is a miserable neurotic. Without defenses we would feel much too vulnerable and scared to venture out into the world and would constantly feel overwhelmed by the actions of others and emotionally bruised. These defenses are learned in childhood, taught perhaps by observing family members who use rants or regression or one of dozens of other defenses to cope with anxiety and frustration. Sometimes these mechanisms have to be taught at a later date in life within psychotherapy. A therapist would like to see a client learn how to blame another as a defense mechanism instead of suffering in a perpetual state of feeling unworthy and weak.

Ego psychologists are interested in how one develops an ego, how one learns to defend one's ego, and how one learns to share those kinds of ego places, that is, one's self with another. French psychoanalyst Didier Anzieu, an ego psychologist, wrote that the ego is inherently linked to skin and that it is through the infant's experience of its skin in contact with others through the act of feeding and nurturing and physically being in skin-to-skin contact with others that teaches the baby its first knowledge of ego.

So, how do we developmentally learn how to use our skin, to get in the skin of another, to make contact with another, or, if we are lucky, to rub someone the right way? The skin is the most remarkable of our sensory organs. It is the only sensory organ that we cannot live without—seeing, hearing, smelling, and tasting are each optional. The skin's biological functions are many: it "breathes and perspires, secretes, and expels, maintains the tonus, stimulates respiration, circulation, digestion, excretion, and of course, reproduction."[20] The skin itself is comprised of three layers: the outer surface is called the epidermis. This self-replacing layer offers protection against scrapes and can both stretch to accommodate movements and then retract to its previous form. The next inner layer, the dermis, provides the skin with elasticity and astonishing toughness; tanned leather is essentially the dermis. The dermis is a network of nerve endings and blood vessels. In addition, the skin is covered in hair, in fact humans have as much hair as primates such as apes, but our hair is much thinner and except for our heads much shorter; therefore we appear less hairy.[21] Consider some of the complexities of skin. We can swim for long periods of time, yet our skin will not fill up with water. Conversely we can drink a gallon of water, and it will not leak out of our pores. Human skin has an ability to stretch dramatically and just as dramatically to shrink. Consider the remarkable fact that a pregnant belly will shrink and return approximately close to its previous size. If skin is flayed from the body entirely, it shrinks up entirely. The skin also has acoustical properties, such as the sensitivity of the skin to vibration, providing hearing-like abilities. The skin also possesses spatial vision-like abilities: think of reading in Braille. In this light, it becomes more apparent how vital the skin is—always alive with sensory capacity, always ready to fill in for the other senses if one should fail. The skin can, if needed, perform seeing and hearing functions in the event that they should be compromised or lost, although the replacement occurs in some mediated fashion. However, there is not anything, not the eyes, nose, or ears, that can replace the function of the skin. The skin stands alone and without it we die.

In Jonathan Cole's book *About Face,* he interviews people who went blind in their adult years. The interviews reveal a complex transition from sightedness into blindness and help to illustrate just how well the skin can contribute to the sense of sight if vision is lost. Much of what we learn through the stories that Cole tells is how emotionally painful it is to lose one's vision after having lead a long life of normal sight. Perhaps the most moving of the intriguing stories told by his interviewees is their descriptions of how, despite their best efforts, eventually they lose the image of familiar faces—even of those most cherished and loved people in their lives. One of Cole's subjects called Jeremy did have facial memories but was unable to control when or who appeared. Seemingly out of nowhere a face from his childhood would appear. Another interviewee named Peter did not experience uncontrollable facial memories, but rather described his heroic effort to retain a kind of portrait gallery of faces. After he realized that his fading vision was irreversible, he swore to himself that even if he lost the images of his friends, he would retain a visual depiction of his wife and children. Unfortunately and to his great dismay, even they began to fade and were eventually lost. Soon after, however, he discovered with great hope that "all the emotion that is in the face is also in their voice. Intelligence, color, light and shade, melody, humor, grace, accuracy, laziness, carelessness, monotony...."[22] This acoustic ability is highly important and enriching, enabling him to communicate and enjoy his social world in a way that is deep and rewarding. If asked whether one would prefer to lose the sense of vision or the sense of hearing, most people would say that they would like to lose their sense of hearing. There is just something instinctual about this response it seems. However, research has suggested that deafness has been shown to leave individuals with a heavy sense of social isolation. The hard of hearing often feel excluded from joining conversations and are not invited by others to participate in social activities, and when they are included, they are unsure of the nuanced meanings of a social exchange often braided into spoken language, such as sarcasm, humor, and emphasis.

At first glance, the heavy influence on the pleasures of hearing in Cole's interviews does not support the idea that tactile sensations play a very important role as a substitute for vision, but what soon emerges is that the skin indeed does play an extremely important role for these visually impaired men. In fact, the role is so important and complex in the way that it supplants visual memories, that it is responsible for becoming it own kind of vision. In these reports, for example, one interviewee tries to explain that what one looks like and what one "looks" like through touching are two very different experiences. "What does continually strike me is the lack of commensurability between what it looks like and what it feels like."[23] He continues to explain the experience of touching the face of his sleeping young son and how moved he is by all the "facial" geography he travels, the "nobs and little bits and pieces. It's a curious tactile thing that I don't think I ever enjoyed as a sighted person."[24] Here, the sense of touch is unlike acoustic stimulation, which has already been well established as a form of sensing and continues to serve in this function after losing sight, if perhaps in a more augmented form. It cannot be said the ears have acquired sight per se. Yet, here we have evidence that the skin has, rather slowly, developed into a seeing organ that was not present before blindness. There is not just amplified touching, feeling more sensitively, because the ears seem to hear more sensitively, but actually seeing by perceiving the world in a new way that gives those who have lost their vision a connection to the world of sight.

At a sociocultural level, the skin factors into many aspects of our relations to one another. It is arguably the way we even manage to recognize one another by identifying acquaintances by their skin. "These characteristics include pigmentation, folds, wrinkles, furrows, the pattern of pores, hair, nails, scars, spots and moles, not to mention the texture of the skin, its scent…, its softness or roughness."[25] Beyond biology, there is much cultural complexity to skin. Consider societies where mothers keep babies closely strapped to their bare backs and others where skin distance is preferred. There are cultures that cut or even mutilate the skin of their children or have ritual, and of course, decorative tattooing.[26]

Arguably, no other psychologist has changed the way we understand the skin as has French psychoanalyst D. Anzieu. Anzieu introduced the psychoanalytic concept of the "skin ego." He defined the skin ego as "a mental image of which the Ego of the child makes use during the early phases of its development to represent itself as an Ego containing psychical contents, on the basis of its experience of the surface of the body."[27] All infants are born into a kind of semi-autistic state where they are fused with the mother. Contained within a kind of mother psychic embryo, newborns and very small infants cannot distinguish between themselves and others. Virtually complete lack of body control ensures that newborns experience their bodies along a shared route of temporarily borrowing the physical attributes of a more developed being to prop them up and provide them with a sense of coordination and movement. After all, what soothes a baby most besides sucking, are externally provided rhythmic movements. Rocking or gentle bouncing are perhaps reassuring at a neurological level, but also at a psychological one in that it provides through the comfort of merger the illusion of coordination and perhaps even a very early sense of effectiveness and identity. Beyond that, all parents quickly learn that the opposite is also effective, that is, being tightly bound up and swaddled. This binding still provides an outside of the self-imposed sense of coordination by preventing the natural little herky-jerky movements all infants display.

Thus, we are all born autistic, in the sense that we live in another world. Freud referred to this state as a type of "oceanic oneness" with the mother.[28] In fact, it was not until about six months of age that ego psycho-analyst Margaret Mahler suggested that the infant psychologically "hatches" and starts taking the small psychic steps toward becoming aware that I am not actually you, but actually a physically and psychically indi-viduated self.[29] These small movements into selfhood, that is, hatching, can first be observed when a baby begins to push off of the mother's skin, gaining distance and a new vantage point. Their bodies begin to permit novel perspectives, and infants will begin to pull another's hair or explore another's face with their hands. Infants during this stage even look differ-ent, more wide-eyed and, well, frankly, as if they have just been hatched. If psychic merger is the first prephase of skin ego development, then the next phase is "the suppression of the common skin and recognition that each has his or her own skin, his or her own skin ego, a recognition which does not come about without resistance and pain."[30]

SKIN AS COMMUNICATION

The remainder of this section is divided into four sections, each examining skin ego functions and their relationship to face transplantation. First, how do we learn to live in our own skin and learn to realize its communicative functions: to listen to one's own self, smell one's own odors, and touch and investigate one's own body by sucking on fingers and toes? Second, once a young child realizes that not only are they capable of using their skin for communication, they must learn that they are a separate being from their mothering caregivers; this process is gradual and involves rituals of hellos and goodbyes and even minor wounding and repair of the skin. Third, chil-dren must learn to contain what is theirs, to keep themselves together and prevent their psychic selves from escaping through psychic pores and open-ings. Finally, antipsychotic functions of the skin ego are discussed whereby re-merging with the maternal skin is avoided and psychosis prevented.

Adam Phillips, in his book *On Kissing, Tickling, and Being Bored*, talks about how we cannot tickle ourselves. Why might be that so? Perhaps if we could tickle ourselves, it would limit our abilities to explore our own bodies. Imagine how much less self-touching and exploration would occur if we experienced our own touches as ticklish! Phillips' thoughts contribute to our understanding of how the skin serves as a psychic communicative conduit between us and others. It is precisely the "me, not me" aspect of the skin that functions with the tickling; that is, I know where I am ticklish, but I cannot tickle myself, the knowledge only makes sense as something that you can find out by touching me: communicating with me. In fact, I could tell you or I could choose not to tell you the special places that make me giggle. Clearly, for the child, a psychosexual precursor of how to explore another's body and for another to explore their own body is to explore pleasure, but initially this is an "enacted recognition of the other."[31] Enacted, because after all, where we are ticklish is rarely one of the later erotogenic zones, thus using the skin to learn how to find places of pleasure, to use the skin of another as a map, is first played out through tickling. The lesson thus becomes one of learning what brings you pleasure: what parts of your body make you smile and laugh. How can I illicit your positive responses? Tickling is also the introduction for the child to discover the line between pleasure and pain, where one becomes aware of how tickling has the potential to become painful and sadistic. Therefore the child learns that touching sensitive parts of another's body brings intense joy, but can also cause pain if over-stimulated: a lesson in how to listen and make adjustments in one's delivery of touches in regards to another's response.

Skinned Separation

Maternal attention for the many little abrasions small children inevitably receive in the form of scraped knees and bloodied elbows offers constant practice at working through what Anzieu refers to as issues of psychically primitive fusing. At an unconscious level, separating from the mother is equated with "the rending of the common skin."[32] We may begin our psychic lives fused with another; however, it is our psychic destiny to work through issues of separation from the mother's corporal self. Each small skin lesion a young child acquires inevitably evokes the maternal/infant shared skin story that follows: to separate from my mother's skin is painful and accomplished with a certain psychic pain, but if we practice this dance of separation and reunion, the boundary between us will become more real and will promote my psychic independence, confidence, and emotional health. Mothering contributes to the dance via both by taking care of a wound with a bandage but also, at least the fantasized potential, with the intention to presently pull the bandages off. After all, the application of every bandage implies that it will soon have to be removed. In fact, beyond their ability to act out psychic renting, bandages are rather useless, offering only minimal protection and coverage and only haphazard coverage at that. Yet little children seem to be stuck on them and are soothed by the ritual application and presumably the painful removal.

In the classic San Francisco–based film noir *Dark Passage*,[33] Lauren Bacall asks Bogie if he would like her to remove the bandage covering his postoperative face in "one short shriek?" Simply put and familiar enough perhaps, it is an intriguing question and illuminates some of the nuances of how those who are mothering assist little children to separate from them by not only attending to scrapes but by subtly damaging the skin through bandage pulling. Anyone responsible for removing a bandage enters Bacall territory, and her question is a familiar one: do you prefer a slow ripping of the adhesive or one short shriek? Ultimately, it does not matter because both methods are painful, and ironically most adhesive bandages produce some minor skin irritation as they lift off hair and small pieces of skin or leave traces of irritation from the adhesive itself. The question of bandage removal is interesting, in and of itself, and hints at a warning that what I am about to do to you is going to hurt and that because I am the one asking the question I am bringing attention to the fact that I am the one who inflicts this pain, not the bandage itself, but my method of removal. Thus, in this ritual, mother both cares for the hurt and then re-hurts the wound—healing and bonding, followed by renting and skin separation, a Seussian-like physical rehearsal of oneness and two-ness, me-ness and you-ness.

The face transplant recipients are told that their transplants could at any time, regardless of how well they have done in the past, still be rejected by the body. The threat of rejection is related to the renting off of maternal skin. The premature symbolic rupture from mothering could potentially put patients into some kind of chronic state of anxiety. Perhaps this worry could even translate into a masochistic hysteric phase where one would unconsciously wish for the transplanted tissue to be voided. From this perspective, it is very possible to understand Clint Hallam wanting to remove his transplanted hand and the man from China having his transplanted penis removed.

Skin-Tainment

Anzieu explains that "as the skin serves as a support for the skeletons and muscles, the skin ego plays the role of maintaining the psyche."[34] Like an invisible envelope, the skin ego holds in fantasy and impulsive behaviors, preventing the more primitive parts of one's psychic being from leaking out. Initially, of course, the function of holding is literally about holding, i.e., mother's hands propping up the baby, and later these hands become psychic hands where the older baby and child can "cling" to these initial physical manifestations to support their independent and "primary identification with a supporting object."[35]

A primary skin ego function is the job of containment. Anzieu's logic is such that the skin ego cannot be a container unless it has something to contain. Here he turns to Freud's conception of the id. What the container is meant to hold inside are id-like impulses that demand attention and are comprised of orality, aggression, and pleasure seeking. As adults, we all have id impulses; they are according to Freud unconscious and difficult to describe because they are also preverbal. Evidence of the id could be heard in Freud's psychoanalytic patients through their slips of the tongue, spontaneous expressions of aggression, and pleasure seeking. We experience the id as a kind of pulsating need machine that lies under the surface. Our ability to contain these raw drives separates us from babies and animals who live out their id impulses.

In Anzieu's conception the skin, ego becomes the "shell," and the inner world of the id becomes the "kernel." Pulsating drives will keep expanding, pouring and stretching out if there is nothing to contain or localize or diffuse them. Imagine if all of our infantile impulses were released and experienced at one time, all of our most elemental urges, fears, and primitive needs escaped. While this catastrophic collapse is unlikely to occur, Anzieu describes what even a partial breach in the kernel might entail and the subsequent psychological consequences. Specifically, he speaks of two forms of anxiety. The first form of anxiety is a kernel with a disrupted sense of shell, creating a diffuse, nonlocalizable anxiety where the person "wraps himself in suffering" in order to form a containment barrier.[36] Created by the loss of a maternal protective shield, a second form of anxiety is initiated where the shell itself is filled with holes, where energy, memories, thoughts, and even the ability to create aggression for self-protection leaks out, or by infantile fears of the fused mother being abruptly torn off, creating imagined holes or ruptures in the primitive skin ego.

Both of these forms of anxiety may be related to face transplantation. First, to have an injured or disfigured face that is removed and replaced by another necessitates the sewing on of skin and the constant threat of tissue rejection. The threat of rejection is the fear of the facial skin developing points of rejected tissue where the skin is weakened and dying, opening up the dreaded holes that leak the very energy that the skin ego aims to contain: a kernel with an insufficient container.

Bodyworlds

The art of von Hagens exhibited in *Body Worlds* (Gunther von Hagens' *Body Worlds: The Original Exhibition of Real Human Bodies* 2006–2007) is interesting in light of the kernel/shell relationship and illustrates what is at risk when the id kernel is exposed and unrestrained. The anatomical art plays a bit of a psychic trick by completely eliminating the actual shell and exposing the kernel, not just the muscles and skeleton in a passive form, but in all of its id-pulsating glory, or perhaps gory. What is fascinating about his work is the way in which he molds the very energy functions into the bodies. They are playing sports and are in poses of running, which ultimately both thrills us (by reassuring us that id energy is indeed organized and not just pouring out) and appalls us (because to see this kernel is forbidden and dangerous).

For the face transplant patient, the possibility of what is at play is the threat of leaking—again the real possibility of the face being rejected bit by bit—therefore evoking unconscious anxieties related to losing oneself and the escape of one's psychic energy. Recall the free associative study in Chapter 2, whereby students wrote group stories on the topic of face transplantation. In those narratives, there was a large amount of violence in the fantasy material, for example, related to the transplant recipient's being attacked or hit by buses. How better to cope with the fantasized fear of the kernel becoming exposed than to fantasize how one must defend oneself from retaliators. Here we may also understand why there are so many references to animals in the fantasy stories; in fact, many of the stories have to do with oral aggression and biting, the most primitive and dangerous type of infantile aggression.

Perhaps the aggression is related to fears of not having aggression, of exposing a psychic inability to defend herself, which highlights the fact that, in the fantasy stories, she has been compromised to the extent that she seems a victim and helpless—a kind of cloak of suffering, one entirely without a kernel. The mother, for Anzieu, provides the infant with a protective mothering skin shield, without the protective layer, or an incomplete one; there may develop a paranoid anxiety that others can penetrate the shield by stealing one's thoughts, or putting thoughts into one's head.[36] Ironically, this lack of protective layer develops when too good of care is given, when one only has had the experience of the protective mothering shield and has not had the opportunity to psychically achieved self-support. Consequently, Anzieu suggests that individuals in that situation may try to protect their egos with a self-made shield of drugs or smoking as a barrier "between the Ego and external stimuli."[37]

Of course, one of the mysteries to Dinoire's doctors was her insistence on smoking so soon after her operation. Now, granted, she was a smoker before the operation, but it is of interest that two of the films concerned with facial surgery share a feature—in both *Dark Passage* and *The Face of Another*, the characters smoke cigarettes through cracks in the bandages over their faces. Certainly smoking in films was historically commonplace; however, in light of Anzieu's theory, that when one does not have a protective shield one may envelope oneself in a smoky layer of protection, considering the actions of these characters, and perhaps of Dinoire, one would assume that having no face or a face of another would lead to such disturbances of safety. Here we may also gain insight into the masks and superhero characters that crowd the collective fantasy stories. Masks here may be another way to create a protective layer, to replace that which has been lost or the fear that it was never developed.

Skin as Barrier

Finally, Anzieu speaks of the skin ego maintaining a sense of boundary and keeping one from falling into Freud's state of the uncanny, where there is "a threat to the individuality of the self through a weakening of its sense of boundaries."[38] Anzieu reminds us that very real problem with transplanted skin is that our bodies are rigged to reject foreign tissue, something he relates as an "anti-function" of the skin.[39] Built into the skin at the cellular level is a message that one's self is not the other and, when the body senses that it has become the other, it will proceed to attack it. This kind of rejecting function is vital in understanding the very real threat of physical tissue rejection and also from a psychological viewpoint, that face transplant recipient's struggle with maintaining a sense of identity. Here we have the ultimate dilemma of identity, where one part of the face psychologically rejects the transplanted section. If the skin ego is there to reinforce the boundaries between two people, then wearing the face of another becomes highly problematic because of the very nature of the procedure that collapses two faces into one. In fact, in the fantasy stories all types of boundaries fail, e.g., the boundary between male and female, the usual sexual boundaries between people, and the boundaries between human and inhuman forms. In the few interviews that have taken place with Dinoire, she does mention her thoughts about boundaries, vis-à-vis identity. For example, she has been quoted as saying, "it will never be me" and "as for this face ... it's not me," she told *Le Monde*. "It will never be me.... A part of me and my identity disappeared forever. And I have precious memories of what I was."[40] Even around the third anniversary of her transplant, Isabelle Dinoire still seems to struggle with her identity. Asked by a French television reporter if she experienced her face as her own or as someone else's, Dinoire responded "it's someone else's. Well it's not the ..., it's not her [the donor], it's not me, it's another face."[41] The uncanny is difficult to resolve.

Perhaps when we say to another, "try to contain yourself," we are trying to help someone to leave a kind of psychotic-like place where they merge with another person or thing. They cannot find their own skin. Michael Eigen's work, as inspired by Bion and Winnicott and outlined in his book *The Psychoanalytic Mystic*, talks about how close we can be to disintegration and psychosis as we retreat to, or become reenveloped with, infantile skin.[42] We may become thin-skinned and vulnerable to psychic shadows and big others that subsume ourselves, smothering and rendering us merged and infantile-like. "We know we are the kind of beings who *can* disintegrate. We step between disintegration threats like children stepping between cracks in the sidewalk, hoping to avoid fault lines of personality."[43]

CONCLUSION

From a culture of narcissism to the skin as psychic boundary between individuals, this first part "Analyzing the Face," Chapter 3 has explored identity and face transplantation through the lens of object relations and ego theory. In Part II in Chapter 4 we enter the worlds of Sigmund Freud and Jacques Lacan, where topics from mystic writing pads to mirrors are explained and creatively connected to the topic of identity and face transplantation.

4

Analyzing the Face: Part II

Many months after news broke to the world of Isabelle Dinoire's face transplant procedure, Dinoire shared a rather startling sentiment with the French newspaper *Le Monde*. After mass media outlets had been furnished with photos of Dinoire's face at different stages of recovery as part of a hospital public relations campaign,[1] Dinoire boldly claimed that, although forever grateful for the new face French surgeons had delivered unto her, "it [the face] will never be me."[2] After all of the media fanfare that followed Dinoire's transplant, including proclamations over the perfection of her healing face by lead transplant surgeon Jean-Michel Dubernard,[3] Dinoire's confession was not only surprising, it was a bit shocking. If Dinoire's procedure had been as successful as surgeons described it to be, from where did her wistful elegy to her "self" emanate?

Much more than simple regret in Dinoire's pensive remark, there is a clear sense of a haunting. This haunting, as is the case with any spectral presence, is a difficult feeling to grasp, yielding only the diaphanous and elusive feeling of being burdened by some force from the past. When confronted with an image of her "new self" as embodied through her face, Dinoire's statement seems to imply that she feels not alone, as though quivering beside her was some dim image of herself as she was before her face transplant. Much speculation has gone into the way that having the face of another deceased human being might haunt a person such as Dinoire in the case of a face transplant. And yet, what Dinoire's case shows is that one of the major psychological obstacles to accepting a new person's face is not the ghost of another person, but the ghost of one's own past. What is the imageless apparition that seems to stand with Dinoire, shoulder to shoulder, in that confrontation if not simply her past? "As for this face ... it's not me," Dinoire told *Le Monde*, "it will never be me ... a part of me and my identity disappeared forever. And I have precious memories of what I was."[4] At the moment Dinoire gained a new face, she likely arrived at a crisis point: she became unable to synthesize her new face into a continuous and cohesive sense of identity that was able to encompass her experiences with both her old and new faces. Surely her identity is more expansive than her face, and yet the loss of her old face has caused a crisis in the flow of her life, in the security of her identity. In some fashion, it seems that the self with which she identified remained attached to the past and was still in the process of expanding to include her new face. Although Dinoire makes it clear that her new face will never be "her," as if to proclaim the incommensurability between her new face and her self, how is it possible to account for this seeming chasm between one's past and future selves?

In Kobo Abe's *The Face of Another* (a novel that is different enough from its film adaptation already mentioned in this work as to merit mention again), the main character, a chemist (as in the film), is badly injured in a chemical accident, leaving his face disfigured. As a result of his injuries, the chemist goes to extreme measures to evade the disgust, scorn, and scrutiny of the everyday encounter with the perception of others that makes him feel like a monster. When the enervating distance of alienation the chemist feels with his wife due to his disfigurement grows unbearable, he designs and creates a realistic-looking mask, a new face in which lies the possibility of a new appearance, an appearance in which he would escape the gaze of other people—including his wife—that makes him *feel* his disfigurement. As the chemist begins to try out his new mask in public, he is alarmed at the positive response he receives from other people. Acting as a man quite unlike his old self, the chemist eventually prefers the personality that burgeons from his use of the mask to his own. And yet, in spite of a return to a normal public life through the use of this mask, the chemist feels plagued by what he once was, especially in his disintegrated relationship with his wife. Resentment toward the lost love of his wife further ferments for the chemist, leading him to devise a plan in which, as his new masked self, he would seduce, ensnare, and eventually exact revenge upon his wife.

In the course of his self-designed and self-inflicted psychodrama, the chemist's incomplete redefinition of himself drives the book to its dramatic climax, where, as the chemist is set to confront and kill his wife, he realizes how far his new face seems to have taken him away from his past. Driven by the painful memories of his old life, the chemist becomes unable to redefine himself through the use of his mask because the mask is merely a smoke screen from having to confront the painful disintegration of his marriage. Even with a new face, a trace of the man's identity, as bound to his happy marriage to his wife, remained and persisted under the surface of his mask persona. Under this mask was an anchor to the past that, the further and harder the man tried to run, tugged tightly on his soul preventing him from ever truly moving forward with his life. With the flourish of many a *noir* tale, Abe's novel charts the classic story of a man on the run from himself, unable to escape the events of his past. Stranded on an island afloat somewhere between the life he had once had and the life he now must live, the chemist lives a life kept frozen in time by the facts of the past that he is unable to move beyond.

Unable to undertake the difficult process of synthesizing traumatic changes and disruptions to one's life within the continuous narrative of one's life, the chemist in Abe's novel forsakes his past in the most peculiar of ways—aiming to recapture it by exacting revenge upon it. Much more than simply "moving on," the psychological struggle in Abe's novel is about the problems that being haunted by one's past creates when the past is the last place a person wants to be. This point, made more apparent in Abe's novel than in Teshigahara's film, is that the loss of one's identity occurs through the experience of becoming dissociated from the past, a problem of experiencing life in continuity with itself. As we see in *The Face of Another*, continuity, as such, is disrupted the moment one tries to escape the past, either through clinging to it, attempting to recapture it, or desperately fleeing from it; even so, the direction one attempts to take to preserve the cherished image of one's past is never lucid; one never has a clear sense of direction, so to speak, when attempting to escape one's past. Without the past you are blind to the future. There is no such thing as a clean break or a fresh start in matters of love and identity.

South Korean "bad boy" director Kim Ki-Duk's film *Time* (2007), a perverse fable about identity, love, and plastic surgery, explores the idea that no matter at what speed a person moves into the future, their past is never far behind. Part romance, part horror (as all of Kim Ki-Duk's films tend to be), *Time* follows a woman, Seh-hee. Long distrustful of her boyfriend's love, Seh-hee hatches and executes a plan to recapture her boyfriend's love and attention anew by transforming her appearance through plastic surgery. Convinced that her looks no longer excite her boyfriend, Ji-woo, Seh-hee disappears from his life and enlists the services of a plastic surgeon in order to completely transform her appearance. Devastated by the sudden and complete vanishing of his girlfriend, Ji-woo remains intentionally impervious to other women, convinced that Seh-hee will one day return to him. When Seh-hee's return begins to seem more and more unlikely to Ji-woo, he slowly emerges from depression and withdrawal and begins to date new women, only to have each romantic encounter broken up at crucial moments by strange interruptions—interruptions the viewer understands as somehow emanating from Seh-hee.

Eventually, however, Ji-woo does kindle a new romance with a woman who seems uncannily familiar to him. Slowly, as Ji-woo's relationship develops with his new love see-hee, the viewer realizes that this woman is actually his old lover—Seh-hee, at the end of surgical transformation. Although Ji-woo's new-found love seems to have allowed him to emerge from the desolation that Seh-hee's disappearance had left him in, elements of See-hee grow increasingly suspicious to Ji-woo: who is See-hee? What is See-hee's past? Where does she come from? Eventually, this enigma becomes clear to Ji-woo, and he is overcome by shock: See-hee is his former lover, Seh-hee. As the film spirals toward its inevitable tragic end, Ji-woo too changes his appearance through the knife of the same plastic surgeon that turned Seh-hee into See-hee. At the film's unexpected and gruesome end, Seh-hee/See-hee runs after a man she believes to be Ji-woo until he is accidentally run over by a car, mutilating his face, and killing him. Because Seh-hee/See-hee had yet to find the new Ji-woo, she is left unable to confirm whether or not the man that was run over by the car was Ji-woo. Even if his face had been left untouched, Seh-hee/See-hee would never be able to tell if it had been Ji-woo.

In a fashion similar to the demented pursuit of the past that we find in *The Face of Another*, the characters of *Time* follow the path of a misguided and misdirected quarry into their past. Rather than entering their past as a means to emerge in an unfolding and open future, they forever seek refuge from the pain of the past by attempting to reenact the past. However, instead of escaping that pain, the characters only end up spiraling out in the vortex of the past.

The title of the film, *Time*, speaks to the sadness of nostalgia that pervades the whole film, driving every decision of the film, including the characters' resolve to transform their identities. The melancholic sentiment to get back to the past, although emanating from within history, is a sure symptom of an occluded movement in time. Unable to recapture the past through the frenzy of metamorphosis, *Time* highlights the very problem *The Face of Another* deals with: how does one find continuity with the past, and in turn, with the self? In this assortment of characters harried by their pasts, their bold moves forward to acquire new faces only make them run into their past in even more violent and jarring ways than they had before donning their new faces. In the jarring encounter with the past, one slowly realizes that identity has less to do with one's face and somehow simultaneously more to do with than one's face than had been previously conceived. The face no longer serves as a sign of identity, but some sort of powerful conduit, the literal loss of which stirs up dramatic and powerful feelings of loss, memory, and the passage of time.

How much of ourselves is tethered to the past? How much of oneself is it possible to abscond with from the past? These questions, although not immediately obvious, are salient issues to be pondered in the context of a face transplant; for face transplants not only provoke the question of an individual person's identity in history, they provoke anxiety over and pose a considerable challenge to the historical model of people speaking about identity.

What is the psychological history of one's identity?

FORWARD INTO THE PAST

Wrestling with the psychoanalytic heritage of an ego-bound individual is one of the long shadows of Sigmund Freud's impact on mass psychology that continued while the practice of psychoanalysis has in recent decades entered a period of gloaming in scientific communities as well as popular public opinion. Although problems with psychoanalysis abound in the world today—and these are arguments that are of no interest to us here— there are excellent preliminary hints in psychoanalytic theory at to how to pursue identity *beyond* the face; going skin-deep with the concept of identity, penetrating the face, and eventually to return back to it, one begins to examine the formation and material of identity.

The commonly accepted launch point of one's conscious psychological life descends from Freud's theory of castration. The problem of castration in psychoanalysis is a tricky one. Vociferously attacked in critiques of psychoanalysis, as well as being the topic of frequent debate in psychoanalytic circles, its seminal status in the developmental lives of individual humans is ponderous and often unclear. As a primordial trauma and prime mover in the psychological development of human beings, castration serves as a considerable force. Without launching into debates on various fronts that contest the accuracy of the theory of castration[5] and avoiding the anatomical implications of the theory, our aim here is to look at the ways in which the experience of castration interacts with the spectral past of a person's sense of self. With our stated interest as such, rather than settling into too many theoretical entanglements, we approach the theory of castration impressionistically, as the moment in which a cut *into* individual identity occurs.

When Freud parses out a discussion of castration in *Totem and Taboo,*[6] he situates castration in relation to the formation of one's face and identity by linking the experience and fear of castration to the process of coming under the influence of the totemic father. It is in relation to the faces in one's family that one gains a face of one's own. Without delving into the anthropological vicissitudes of Freud's understanding of castration, suffice it to say that Freud was after developing a theory of how it is that humans come to acquire a proper name and inherit the cultural marks of their predecessors and how identity becomes solidified. Many elements play into the rather complex process of castration, much more than a simple experience of becoming aware of the vulnerability of one's human anatomy, including the awareness of the existence of entities in the world as being separate from oneself and command over language acquired through learning the process of naming the things in one's environment—including oneself. This is the world that the child gains through the sacrifice of one's early childhood created by castration.

The venture of childhood is marked by the joyful babble of growth, but is also is permeated by the pain of what it means to grow: to let go. What is referred to as castration anxiety, although understood in many different ways, is perhaps best explained by understanding that it has less to do with a fear of the past, of the traumatic event of castration, as the fear of a new move into the future created by the cut of anxiety. Any such new move necessarily demands a letting go—the experience on which all fear in castration anxiety is focused. The problem with any such obligatory movement forward falls back to the very problem Freud's patient Dora encountered in her own experience of losing face in regard to her father. Asking Dora's question "who and what am I?" is the dawning of the dread that one experiences when confronted with the experience of losing face. As the writer Elias Canetti says in a discussion of totem power from his monumental work of social psychology, *Crowds and Power,* "the mask is clear and certain, but is loaded with the terror of uncertainty. Its power derives from the fact that it is itself known, while what it covers is never known. The mask is only known from outside or, as it were, from in front."[7] Canetti here describes the totemic fear involved with losing one's face, not unlike the experience Dora went through, which was, in ways, the experience of becoming ashamed of her father, watching the totem mask be ripped off of her father's face. But what is it that lies underneath that face? The answer in psychoanalytic terms can provide a simple enough and obvious answer: one's unconscious past; but what does that mean and what does one do with it? As some sort of disturbing and chaotic force, bubbling beneath one's face, the disturbing nature of the past—as a haunting—is inchoate and unclear. What is it then that people fear behind the mask? As novelist

Alexander Theroux wonders of the dark side of human beings, "do we fear the Gorgon or simply create it to locate our fears?"[8]

An unlikely but relevant place to begin our examination of a psychoanalytic understanding of identity and its past can be found in an obscure little essay by Sigmund Freud, one of the few essays he ever authored that focused on popular culture, "The Mystic Writing Pad."[9] Although ostensibly a meditation on the functions of the human mind in its unconscious and conscious forms, Freud's essay evokes an interesting way of thinking about the *layers* of a person, in terms of the affective interaction of one's physiology, the conduct of one's sense of self, the sedimentation of meaning in a life, and, through an understanding of memory, the chronological formation of subjectivity. In this essay, Freud describes a newly released children's toy of the 1920s, a writing pad that consisted of a layer of cellulose, a layer of waxed paper, and a bottom layer of resin or wax. On the surface, Freud's reading seems to be a routine reading of a metaphor for consciousness: writing layers on top = conscious, bottom wax slab = unconscious. However, when one inspects this short essay more closely, it is startling to notice that what Freud seems to be addressing is the relationship between the production of psychical energy and the formation of the mind's boundaries and the way in which sensual tendrils facilitate this relationship. In part, the mystic writing pad was an attempt to mine out the charge of memory as the binding agent that interacts between unconscious and conscious worlds.

According to Freud's reading of the toy, we possess a system, Pcpt-Cs, which receives perceptions (Pcpt) but retains no permanent trace of them, so that it can react like a clean sheet (Cs) to every new perception, although the permanent traces of the excitation that have been received are preserved in "mnemic systems" lying behind the perceptual system.[10] And that "if we imagine one hand writing upon the surface of the Mystic Writing-Pad while another periodically raises its covering sheet from the wax slab, we shall have a concrete representation of the way in which I tried to picture the functioning of the perceptual apparatus of our mind."[11] The mystic writing pad may appear as a natural example for him to draw on for designating what is usually thought of as the internal/external components of psychical reality; however, the relationship between the two is more oblique than one first may note, perhaps even more complex than even Freud realized.

Far from being simply an impressible surface that contains the traces of all inscriptions, it is the crucial surface, without which writing becomes impossible, and, indeed, on account of which writing on the pad can occur. Conceived along these lines, the wax slab surely interests Freud not only as that which receives the "excitations"[12] of the writing being done on the overlaying pieces of paper, but also for the fact that the excitations of writing, or, perception, are sustained by the underlying wax slab, functioning quite clearly as the unconscious of the slab. The mystic writing pad must have surely summed up for Freud the very way that, contrary to common sense, perception and consciousness are sustained by the unconscious. Here, Freud's interest in the writing pad takes on pretty clear implications of sense, or one could even say, the way tactile sensors play into the question of energy. The question of psychic energy, and especially its relationship to the body, was, if one looks even at Freud's early work on aphasia (at a time when he was still deeply immersed in the problems of neurology), this question of psychic energy is even at play there. Freud's interest in the mystic writing pad as a model of a sort of the psychical function of energy should then be no surprise.

Nevertheless, thinking of the writing pad in this way opens up interesting implications for the psychical functioning of the skin in a way that inverts the traditional understanding of a psychical envelope. What element of the mystic writing pad might we ascribe to the function of the skin? Is it something like the function of an ego, operating as the intelligible, identifiable product of the writing? Here, we are posed with one clear insight from the mystic pad that must be probed further: What is it that remains when the cover is lifted, and what is it that remains that made the cover possible in the first place? What then, if not the obvious? The mark of the past.

Castration is an interesting idea to consider in light of face transplants, precisely through the procedure's relationship to *cuts*. Although there are obvious cuts—losing one's face, gaining a transplanted face, and the reconstructive surgical process made through minor incisions. Following Freud, if castration creates an energy of the self in the form of the unconscious, then what is this energy's relation to the past?

While claiming that she had "returned to the planet of human beings" after receiving her face transplant, Dinoire stated, rather hauntingly that, "a part of me and my identity disappeared forever. And I have precious memories of what I was."[13] One may wonder as to whether Dinoire's words show an ambivalence toward her new face, as well as the presence of some specter. This specter, certainly has the character of the "Mystic Writing Pad" as evoked by Freud, which, although deprived of its external covering, retains the traces of excitations, some leftover energy, enigmatic as it may seem, that powers one's identity. There seems to be something at play in Dinoire's statement that clearly implies a force that outlives the loss of a visible marker of identity, an invisible monument to a sense of self that exists beyond one's appearance.

Cindy Jackson, "The Living Doll,"[14] was a woman who, several decades ago, had felt poorly about her appearance and turned to extreme surgical intervention as a solution. In order to provide herself with an appearance that seemed to match what she deemed to be her "truer" self, Jackson began to undertake a vast number of cosmetic procedures to her face and body in order to provide a truer self that, for Jackson, was trapped within her less-than-thrilling body. But rather than simply touching up little parts of herself that Jackson was unhappy with, her cosmetic ambitions were much more iconic: Cindy Jackson's dozens of procedures were all directed to making her look like Barbie. Although no actual face transplant proper occurred in the case of Cindy Jackson, the sort of surgical-cosmetic self-therapy found in her surgical conquest of low self-esteem exemplifies an almost commonplace and superficial understanding of identity. The naïve and superficial understanding of identity found in Jackson's procedures is symptomatic of a certain way of understanding identity that stands behind the explosive proliferation of cosmetic surgery in the past half century. Although Cindy Jackson has never hinted at any fundamental unhappiness with her new "self" and actually goes on record stating how cosmetic procedures have vastly improved her life, the simple fact that someone like Cindy Jackson routinely subjects herself to plastic surgery, seemingly without end, is enough to point to a deep danger that resides within perpetual self-transformation. The movement of self-transformation is only ever transformative when one is reconciled to what it is they are moving forward from.

What cannot be reconciled to Jackson's new face is, precisely, the uncanny energy related to traces that Freud wrote of in "A Note Upon 'The Mystic Writing-Pad.'" But why should this energy remain inassimilable? What compels someone to put their body through an endless process of body modification without ever arriving at a point of satisfaction? Although Jackson's enjoyment of transformation borders on the pathological, the eager celebration of transforming one's appearance does, in some sense, create a loop of predictability and continuity that, in ways, feels comforting. In so doing, one creates a level of control over their self that never forces a confrontation with aspects of reality that are beyond one's control, for instance, the events of one's past. What radical transformative procedures such as Jackson's ultimately attempt is to circumvent the experience that defines one's identity: being connected to its formation in the past.

MIRROR, MIRROR

In psychoanalysis there is what could be called the "crucial developmental moment," when the child takes a sort of rite of passage from an infantile preconscious state to the state of what one would consider to be that of the language- and symbol-using conscious human. This crucial developmental moment inevitably concerns a separation, a historical division of the child's world into an organized entity wherein the child first perceives itself as being separate from some object, giving birth to the first inklings of a self. In some sense, this is what the French psychoanalyst Jacques Lacan was driving toward with his early essay "The Mirror Stage as Formative of the *I* Function as Revealed in Psychoanalytic Experience."[15] Traditionally conceived as an exposition into the way in which subjectivity is posited through a moment of alienation when one is able to perceive their self as an object through abstraction, resulting in, as Lacan put it, "the finally donned armor of an alienating identity that will mark his entire mental development with its rigid structure."[16] Although "alienating" does indicate the sense in which one is set apart from a world of objects as an individual, there is another sense to the alienated status of the "finally donned armor," as he puts it, of which identity is an upshot. If, in the crucial developmental moment, identity is posited through a hall of mirrors, it is not through the reflection that substantiates identity, but, more precisely, through the aspect of appearance that both eludes and prefigures the specular image of development.

The element that underlies the creation of an abstracted image of what a person is—their identity—is this elusive element. What happens in abstraction, in something like the mirror stage, is the attempt for the child to coordinate its polymorphous needs in order to better acquire them, a process of abstraction that functions, as Lacan points out, "first and foremost like elements of a heraldry, a heraldry of the body."[17] By creating a representation of one's body, a "heraldry," one is able to channel needs and meaning in the world in a more efficient and pleasurable way. In some sense, making the world more comprehensible and graspable is possible only by simplifying one's world—their body—into a simple entity: identity. Unfortunately, the only way this can occur for the child is through a process of abstraction, an act of the representation of need that inevitably fails as the needs of a child are satisfied precisely because they are immediate, and not coordinated through a process of abstraction. The failure of the attempt to coordinate the world into an organized system of sense and meaning is what results in the painful reality of castration for the individual. Rather than immediate needs, the child is left with a method of abstractly constructing its needs, representing needs that are, in a sense, not even there, except in the sense given body by the word that exists through the process of castration. This process of abstractly creating needs is that by which one gains their proper name—the emergence of an identity.

Consider the image of a vampire before a mirror. What we see in the mirror is not the absence of an image, but the presence of some sort of spectral imprint of the body divested of a body. Although the image of a vampire may be somewhat overused in psychoanalytic theory, it takes up Freud's idea of an energy of the past—the product of castration—in an interesting way: rather than mere animating force for an unfolding life, when treated as unconscious and thus remote, this energy takes on a spectral nature—that of a creature of the night. The flesh, the creature of the night that we are left with after castration is something that Lacan designated by the name of a mythical monster-like organ: *lamella*. As the Slovenian philosopher Slavoj Zizek points out, "*lamella*, the 'undead' object, is not a remainder of castration in the sense of a little part which somehow escaped the swipe of castration unscathed, but, literally, the *product* of the cut of castration, the *surplus* generated by it."[18] Imagine an organ, not visible to the eye, but something metaphysical, in a Freudian sense, coating the underside of the skin, penetrating the skin's surface, opening its pores, teasing its follicles, and subjugating its orifices; conceive of this, and this is very much *lamella*. Lamella, this insubstantial organ, somehow acts as the seat of subjectivity, the energy of the past that takes on corporeal form upon which one's identity is hemmed. When the face is lifted back, what remains is not simple flesh, but the traces of the dynamic emergence of identity that bear the historical marks of castration in the form of an unconscious energy of the past.

In order for identity to emerge in childhood, the body must pass through a process of temporal abstraction through castration, an initiation that comes at a price. As one's identity is not formed out of a vacuum, the past from which castration ostensibly separates an individual leaves a certain stain on an individual's life and identity. Approaching the body as if it were stained, the perspective of castration, a cut forms one's face, and one's entire identity springs forth, an unbearable organ of inhuman energy of whose tether to reality is the true horror of the unconscious. The importance of the face, then, would not reside merely in its symbolic function as the linguistic support of one's identity; the importance of the face is to be discovered in the ambivalent feelings one attaches to it as a remnant of the past. In order to imagine the face as such, one must first come to grips with that which finds identity in a face: specters and shame.

GIVING UP THE GHOST

Celebrated German Expressionist director Robert Wiene's film *The Hands of Orlac* (1924; later remade several times, once under a different title and starring Peter Lorre) is a neo-Gothic update of the story of Frankenstein starring Conrad Veidt as the pianist Paul Orlac, a celebrated musician who wrestles with the question, "does the body rule the mind or does the mind rule the body?" after receiving the hands of another man in a transplant procedure. After a train that is bringing the famous pianist Paul Orlac home from a performance derails, Orlac's wife and butler race to the scene of the train's accident and sort through the scene, pulling Orlac's body from the train's wreckage. Scarcely alive, Orlac is rushed immediately to a hospital. A doctor at the hospital informs Orlac's wife that, even though her husband had been brought back from the mortal precipice his injuries had pushed him toward, his hands had sustained severe enough damage as to necessitate their removal.

Bowled over by this news, Orlac's wife desperately exhorts the doctor to do everything in his power to save her husband's hands: the hands of a celebrated musician. The doctor resorts to his only option in the situation: an experimental hand procedure. In the film's Frankenstein-like plot twist, the hands that the doctor uses in his procedure are not the hands of a normal man, but that of a recently executed murderer—a fact that the doctor suppresses from Orlac. Orlac, plagued by visions of enormous spectral hands reaching out for him in his hospital recovery bed, in spite of the doctor's efforts, begins to suspect the abject origins of his new hands, throwing Orlac into terror. Unable to free himself from the possibility that he had received the hands of a cold-blooded murderer—and with them impulses of malevolence—unable to play piano with the fingers of a murderer, Orlac's life begins to spin out of control (a vertiginous plot device we seem to find in many tales of identity crisis), building to the moment that his estranged father is found murdered and the prints from fingertips of Orlac's transplanted hands are found all over the crime scene. Orlac's fate is only saved at the last minute when a woman reveals that the real murderer, a man who had been appearing to Orlac as the phantasm of the executed murderer whose hands Orlac received, was not a phantasm but the murderer of Orlac's father. Intending to frame Orlac for the murder of his father, this man had committed the crime by using wax impressions of the fingerprints of Orlac's new hands, leaving an evidence trail at the crime scene leading back to Orlac. Not only was this man responsible for Orlac's father's death, but he had also framed the executed criminal from whom Orlac's hands had come. In a climactic moment of catharsis, Orlac realizes that the hands he had received in his transplant had, in fact, never been those of a murderer, but of an honest man, unrightfully convicted and executed for the crime of another.

As a perfect compliment to the Frankenstein myth, *The Hands of Orlac* deals with one of the major problems of the story of Frankenstein that is only implied in the myth: the back story of the flesh catching up with its new body—history and the past. Giving new meaning to the experience of phantom limbs and phantom organs (people who experience the back story of their transplanted tissue in the form of also receiving the taste, memories, etc., of another person), *The Hands of Orlac* articulates a plangent point regarding problems of identity: when things don't work out, we blame it on the past. Recall that Clint Hallam, the recipient of the world's first hand transplant procedure, after having his hand removed because it was too psychologically difficult to cope with having a different person's hand, was vilified as an improper candidate for such a procedure because he had been a convicted criminal.[19] But, even before Hallam's criminal past was revealed to the public, the collision of Hallam's past with his new hand was already a concern:

> the patient described phantom-limb sensations of sudden feelings of finger movements, and cramping pain in the hands from time to time, as well a "pins and needles" on exertion of the forearm stump over the past eight years. Since the recipient was able to [play the piano before amputation], he was encouraged to exercise his forearm muscles as if he was playing the piano in preparation for transplantation.[20]

What seems to have been problematic in the case of Clint Hallam was a complete inability to take up the question of his past in any sort of therapeutic fashion. Already hinted at in this quote from Dr. Dubernard is the idea that Hallam does not quite understand that the reception of a new body part, especially one that would impact such an important part of a person's identity (in this case, Hallam identified himself as a pianist). Just as Orlac was able to renarrate the history of his hands at the end of *The Hands of Orlac*, Hallam, and anyone else unable to enter into a new phase of identity, is doomed psychologically to run into a wall. When Hallam's past was blamed by surgeons for his psychological instability in rejecting the transplant, they were not far from the truth. So long as the past is a force that haunts, instead of a force that compels, one's identity and psychological life will remain precarious.

The twisting of the hands of fate that we find in *The Hands of Orlac* begins to offer a different way to think about the psychoanalytic problem of castration; with Orlac, the tale is less about returning to the scene of some sort of trauma that would lead him to believe the fact that he was a criminal, but the problem of incorporation: how does he make sense of the alarming experience of having another person's hand sewn onto his arm? Exceeding its destiny as a myth, the story of *The Hands of Orlac* has come to life in an uncanny way in the form of the world's first double arm transplant, taking place in July 2008 in a hospital in Munich, Germany. The recipient of the procedure, a fifty-four-year-old male patient, had lost both of his arms in a threshing machine accident in 2002, leaving him unable to care for himself in an everyday fashion, a situation that had left him disconsolate and suicidal. In a procedure that involved thirty participants, five surgical teams, and sixteen hours of work, surgeons at the Isar Clinic in Munich transplanted the arms of a recently dead nineteen-year-old Bavarian man onto the body of the fifty-four-year-old man in a complicated procedure that involved not only chilling the transplanted body parts, preserving their blood flow, but also jump-starting blood flow in the arms so that warm blood and not life-threatening cold blood would course through the arms and body of the fifty-four-year-old man.

Some of the connections between this procedure and the film *The Hands of Orlac* should be fairly obvious, but beyond transplanted limbs, the problem of the past, just as it was for Clint Hallam (and someone like Dinoire, as well), rears itself again in this most recent procedure. The transplantation of the arms of a young man onto an old man is not just a logistical problem of making differently aged flesh pair together; as a therapist at Munich University told *The Times*, "this is more than a piece of surgery…the doctors are grafting a completely new identity on this man."[21] Of all of the doctors' caveats that were thrown to this man regarding the issue of receiving the arms of a nineteen-year-old man, including the warning that young arms do not a young man maketh, one lesson should be clear: beware of the insidious appeal of disregarding the past. Although, as it was possible for Orlac, it is possible to take up the past in a new way, it is never possible to rewrite or discard it. The past is defined precisely by what it is not; it's created through displacement; but just because it has come to be, does not mean that it no longer *is*. Just as all other time in a person's life, the past is always changing and is always in flux. Simply disregarding the amazing potential with which the past bears upon one's life is a sure recipe for tragic consequences. Precisely by not being able to change the past, by lacking the possibility of *renarrating* it (in the naïve and relativistic way that Narrative Therapists believe to it be possible), can one truly take up the past, a fecund source for possibility and hope. As Dr. Biemer, the lead surgeon on the double-arm transplant put it in rather Orlacian fashion: "He won't play the piano, but otherwise he will live much better than before."[22] Function and appearance may change, but the past does not. The past only comes to be transformed in the way it is taken up in a story of one's identity as one's life undergoes changes. It is only natural to understand the possibilities of the past to exist and take form as the future lends new perspectives from which to gaze back at it. However, the haunting begins the moment one believes that physical transformation has left the past behind.

If we have the presence of a specter on the one hand, according to psychoanalytic theory, it is the leftover from castration, the organ created by the face, that serves to remind one of the process of castration. In this reminder of castration stands the anxiety that causes the shame of the body, a shame experienced as a concealing agent that, as a reminder, also forces a person to forget and flee their past. This ghostly organ, which pesters and disturbs an individual, is not the problem of being an organ that one cannot incorporate, as Lacanian theory might posit, but the nagging voice of the past that seems to say "don't even try to forget!" The plea of one's past, created by castration, that compels one to cling to their face and identity is a guilt that hectors a person, blocking them from leaving the confines of their past and preventing the immaculate communion with one's self that is required to move on from the fiercely guarded borders of the past. The ghost that harries an individual is never one's true self, offended at the prospect of being forever left behind, but the jealousy of the present that refuses any form of separation from one's past. To relieve oneself of the overwhelming guilt of betrayal of one's past, one must not treat the past as a haunting, but as the force from which one draws new possibilities for the future. And although the psychoanalytic approach to the past does not stand entirely in opposition to this sort of understanding of the past, the language with which psychoanalysis describes the past has become too much a ghost, restricting the possibilities with which one can speak of the past. Possibility does not demand putting the past to rest, for the purpose of putting ghosts to rest it is not enough to tell a new story. To give a new story to a face, one must understand the workings of the narrative of identity, and how the face, a crucial component of such, interacts with other elements of one's appearance, body, and existence.

The many ghosts of how we approach speaking of human beings should not simply be discarded as faulty or wrong, but must be refined and built on. The psychoanalytic understanding of the formation of an individual through the developmental process of castration is not incorrect in the way it models approaching the past; it just does not take the idea of castration far enough. The crucial developmental moment, as an instant of time outside of one's history that reorders it, should be understood as a juncture that human beings are bound to repeat so long as the possibilities of the future remain open. Much like a game of pinball, a person's identity gains a different coordination and direction at each juncture, encountering a series of relative and equally important developmental moments in which the self is always being pulled out of where it finds comfort, into new phases of identity. As such, castration should be understood as the traumatic *cut* that serves as the perfervid force compelling one's life story forward. Dinoire's struggle to find a sense of self in the difficult process of incorporating a new face into one's identity is really no more different than the experience of any person encountering an identity crisis through a traumatic and unprecedented experience. This was the problem that Freud's Dora faced, a problem he was unable to fix for he was too fascinated with the spirits that haunt human beings in the form of the unconscious. To give up the ghost of the unconscious and truly open up new parameters of experience for the afflicted person, we must do away with the humanistic shame that stands in the way of realizing the truly radical insight: that the inhuman mass, the remainder of castration, is the ultimate unique component for every individual and the ultimate condition for allowing one to redefine their experience of the world.

The danger of saying that identity is wholly bound up with appearance is met equally in its ill-conceived vision of identity by another that states that a person is not their face, for both fail to grasp the idea that one's face and one's identity are formed through the forces of time. Age lines, scars, pockmarks—the face contains many traces of the past, the signs of significant events, and begins to become a profound symbol of a person's identity through its temporal formation and not through a denoting or signifying role. Each mark of the face must be regarded not as a phantom at which one will always tremble in silence, but a sign pointing to a new story— reminders of the past that serve as opportunities to transform the past. One's scars can either be symbols of great tragedies, or chances to reimagine the landscape of one's life. Regarding the face as such will inevitably lead to a more dynamic way of talking about identity that makes room for other people within one's skin, exceeding the limits of the story one's identity has thus far proven to be. The more room that is made for meaning in one's skin, in one's face, and in one's identity, leaves less and less opportunity for one to be severed from the past; when it becomes possible to incorporate the past, ghosts are laid to rest.

In place of the time-bounded border that psychoanalysis's investigation of the past places on human beings, we do not suggest that human beings become timeless creatures. Rather, it is important to point out that the function of identity, as oriented by time, must be tracked from the past and into the future—a future that implies new and bold descriptions of what it means to be human. The ghostly past of how we have once understood the boundaries and formation of the identities of individual human beings is the spectral elephant in the operating room of face transplants. The border that face transplant procedures challenge is not merely epidermal; it is the implicit border that informs our ability to speak of all aspects of what it means to be human. Overcoming by exploring what it means to have a past in relation to one's identity allows a new way of approaching the experience of continuity—an experience of time—within the flow of one's identity.

The identity of a person does not simply unfold from one pinprick in the past, gnarling its way forward to the moment in which one presently stands, but is the past, as an open number of moments perpetually colliding with one another in the constant rebirth of what and who a person is. The adventure of the past is merely a loop in the existence of a person, a lap that one must take to bound forward into a development that one's future beckons; to remain mired in the past is to maintain a devotion to a time that is no more responsible for whom a person is than any other time, including (and perhaps, in ways more important) what and when is occurring with a person as they speak. Viewing "who" a person is in this kind of a scattershot temporal fashion not only bypasses the problems of understanding the development of one's identity as the attachment to and the formation of one's face as a linear process, it also allows a person to understand identity as dynamic in a way at which even psychodynamic psychological theories are not quite on par. What is problematic, for example, for Dinoire when she says that her face will never be "her," is not to say that the face transplant procedure has failed to make her new face correspond to a moment of origin in the formation of her identity, but that in her recovery process, there has been a lack of synthesizing therapeutic techniques that would allow her to incorporate the experience of having received the face of another person as part of the narrative of her life. What Dinoire needs is a fuller evocation of what it means to receive the face of another that does not merely embrace the face of another person, but one that learns to embrace her past as a force of potentiality and not as a trammel.

What then is needed is a theory of identity that does not offer a person the possibility of dissembling in the abyss of one's unconscious, avoiding having to moralize what should seem be regarded as a natural expression of existence: in the words of the philosopher Henri Bergson, "I change, then, without ceasing."[23] By treating this statement of Bergson's as descriptive of the natural state of human beings, rather than as situational and exceptional, an evocation of identity as movement versus static entity should become clear. Without refuting the positions of psychoanalysis on the development of personal identity, one can reasonably assert that the development of a procedure such as a face transplant, which gives a new face to the human experience and our understanding of the human being, also demands a new face to how one conceives of identity. In the idea that identity is an entity of flux, rather than an anchor one can situate in the face, its underside, or in conscious and unconscious states, one finds a new psychological approach to talking about identity. This new approach to identity is first formulated by moving beyond static conceptions of identity, through the very question of what roles the past, the face, and all other entities in a person's life play in the story of identity. Such a vision of identity would play host to a way of taking up the past that is both complex, focused on the future while maintaining a sense of purpose in clarifying the problem of the burdens of the past. In order to move on with a discussion of this new face of human boundaries, one must let theoretical ghosts be past without desecration or desertion; although the psychoanalytic understanding of the unconscious spirit of the past takes an exploration of the vicissitudes of one's personality in an important initial direction, the movement is nonetheless incomplete. In order to talk about face transplants and any insights related to identity that emerge from a procedure as unprecedented as face transplants, we must find a new direction in our concepts that does justice to the emergent nature of identity as always in formation and in communication with the past as it forges into the future.

Face transplants inevitably provoke the ghosts of the past that haunt not only how we understand the human body, but our own individual physical histories with our selves, our identities. In eclipsing the apparitional past, one not only foregoes the attachments and feelings he or she has attached to events, others, and their self from the past, they also relinquish the ideas with which they navigate and understand the world in favor of fuller concepts that encapsulate ideas of the past; in place of the old borderland of the human being, face transplant procedures ask humans to conjure a new story for what it means to be a human being—our limits, capacities, future, and past. It is part of the story of identity in which face transplants not only participate but also serve to reveal new directions.

Having traced the contours of the human body and face, psychoanalytic theory seems to point to the past as the dimension of a human being that is most at stake in a face transplant procedure. Following these hints through a historical understanding of identity, face transplants have brought us to a point where we are able to move on from the past, to give up the ghost of ideas that define how we speak of identity, as well as the reality in which human beings are participants. The ghost of the human shell, the one that is difficult to relinquish when we too gladly cling to the past, must too be put to rest, and in its place, a new vision of a human that bears with it a new face— both in understanding and appearance. To move into the next part of the story of identity, of humans, and of face transplants, we must peel back the page that lies before us, growing a new skin in the process, a new face from which to peer that emerges as we tell the tale of a story whose ending we must await. Where next does our tale take us?

5

Narrating the Face

FACES ON FILM

In his seminal essay on film, "The Face of Garbo," literary theorist Roland Barthes succinctly described the uneasy dialectic that seems to reside at the root of all face-identity problems. While charting out a brief history of the cinema up until the 1960s, Barthes points out that the advent of the cinematic medium and the way that it represents human form—referencing the legendary Swedish vixen Greta Garbo and the fawn-like Audrey Hepburn—has had a startling effect on the way we construe human form. For Barthes, the face of Greta Garbo, when viewed on film, represented something of a classical, beatific face, but because of the cinematic representation, says Barthes, "in this deified face, something sharper than a mask is looming."[1] For Barthes, this looming presence was the undoing of a classical representation of beauty, a classical representation that embedded itself in an understanding of the face as a static and unexpressive symbol. Although Garbo's cinematic face began the evolution toward a more complicated facial pattern, the use of cinema was not enough to undo the hegemony of the Ideal face: "the Essence became gradually obscured, progressively veiled with dark glasses, broad hats and exiles: but it never deteriorated."[2]

Nonetheless, Garbo's face represented the point where the cracks made to the traditional conception of a face could no longer be filled in or ignored; Garbo's face represented "... this fragile moment when the cinema is about to draw an existential from an essential beauty, when the archetype leans toward the fascination of mortal faces."[3] In Garbo's face, Barthes saw something of a watershed moment in the crisis of a how the significance of a face is understood, where "an almost unique specification of the face, which has nothing of the essence left in it, but is constituted by an infinite complexity of morphological functions"[4] emerges in the place of fixed face, a mask that serves as the single conduit for construing a person. Somewhere in the history of cinema between Greta Garbo and Audrey Hepburn, Barthes saw a fundamental change in the way faces played expressive roles in films, moving from the firm deified features of ancient bust-portraiture, to expressive ambiguity of da Vinci's all-too-human *Mona Lisa*. Barthes described this fundamental change in the role of the face with the famous line, "the face of Garbo is an Idea, that of Hepburn, an Event."[5] In this historical shift within cinematic representation Barthes sees a face that moves from ideas to events, a shift that we could describe as the gradual descent from a self-identity housed within a mask of ideals to a self-identity defined by multiplicity and possibility. A face construed through multiplicity and possibility—a face closer to the way we experience it everyday—begins to reveal what is problematic about knowing ourselves with simplicity rather than coming to know our identity through the questioning glances of complexity, taking in the full breadth of identity.

The downfall of the classical simplicity of a face, understood as being something more like a mask, did not alone occur through simple technological intervention, but through the fashion in which cinematic technology refined and redefined the function of a face within a story. Early films, largely conceived of as photographic representations of stage dramas, were not quite able to capture the feeling of movement in images that the advent of cinema technology granted. Faces for these early films were like floating paintings from which dialogue emanated. This is the legacy of a classically refined face of an "essence" to which Barthes refers in the example of Garbo. Some early films, however, got the "motion" part of "motion pictures" (such as the comedy films of Mack Sennett that were always centered on the physical comedy), sought to tell stories through the expression of the body, through the movements of motion pictures, granting a new power and expressivity to a face and body robbed of essence. When Barthes refers to Hepburn's face as an "event," he is referring to this expressivity that appreciates the complexity of a face whose Mona Lisa-like ambiguity lends it to possibility and not essential "truth."

Now, one way of taking up this development in cinema is to say that it radically reduced the expression of a person to their face, and perhaps there is some truth to this. However, the other side of the development of a cinematic face was that it developed new expressive capacities for a face, new uses, and new meanings for a face that were not present in classical representations of faces. Overdetermining the face in such a way was achieved by making the face a prominent element in the development of plot, often giving faces their own stories within the larger story of a film. The basis of cinematic storytelling then came to depend not merely on faces, but on the new expressive capacities of faces. One can see this evident in early films such as Carl Theodor Dreyer's *Joan of Arc* (1928) or the innovative technique of sharply zooming in on faces at key dramatic moments found in the gritty films of director Sam Fuller. The face is always the site on which the changes in cinema have taken place, where new technological reflections of reality become convincing (sound emanating from the mouth, the balance of colors on the face, and the stark clarity of features found in digital).

No longer was the face a static, ever seductive visage; the face developed into the most moving of all moving images found on the silver screen. Perhaps cinema created too much of a fascination with faces at the expense of the rest of the human person and the human body. However, the telling of stories through gestures of the body, and then through the effusive gestures of the face, eventually complemented by more and more refined elements of technology and performance created not only new ways in which we perceive the possibilities and capacities of faces, but also a change in the way we perceive our bodies (and our selves) that can be remarkably described in novels such as Adolfo Bioy Casares' *The Invention of Morel* (1940) or J. G. Ballard's *The Atrocity Exhibition* (1970) and in films such as David Cronenberg's *Videodrome* (1983)—all stories heavily concerned with humans interaction with moving images. When technology opens up some new dimension of human experience through questioning our self-conceptions and ideas of the body, the fundamental ways in which we define ourselves as human beings shift. Included in this shift is the way we construe personal identity.

New forms of technology inevitably provoke ambivalence; we have certainly seen this to be case with face transplant procedures. Not only does new technology offer a glimpse of an unknown world, of a great new world of adventure and discovery, but in its movement forward technology demands of people to imagine their world in a new way. This sort of change in a person's world need not necessarily be profound; it only asks of a person to become reconciled to the significance and meaning of the elements that make up their identity. Although we have shown in previous chapters that the idea of a face transplant has captured the imaginations of many through a cinematic representation of the procedure, face transplants, as they relate to self-identity, share much in common with the creation of cinematic narratives. They show that any story, even that of a person's life, is never reducible to one perspective or one simple story.

The problem with any approach to identity that relies on identifying too strongly with a particular part of a person is not that it fails to conceive of a story to that part of the person. What is problematic is the narrow view of just what a story is that one finds in the simplistic understanding of identity: they fail to acknowledge the complex depth and breadth that constitutes a person's identity. The fundamental problem with stories, says the late sociologist Charles Tilly, is that, "even when they convey truths, stories enormously simplify the processes involved."[6]

A face is not a story unto itself, but is a conduit for many tales, a site that merely reflects the presence of many stories and many *times*: marks of long ago, yesterday, and today preside over every face. Faces organize the stories of our lives by making us recognizable, but they can also make us unable to respond to change, and thus, unrecognizable to ourselves. One only need recall Isabelle Dinoire's famous "It's not me" for ample evidence of this fact. There is a larger context to the face wherein an inconceivable number of stories have already taken place, exist, or lie germinating, yet to be told. When we lose sight of this larger context, we run into trouble. But no matter where the storytelling stands in process, one thing is for sure: the story is you, and that story is far more complex than the apparent simplicity with which we wish to tell it.

THE FACE AND THE CROWD

We use our faces to engineer the flow of a complicated and multifaceted world, stories in which our identity not only plays the roles of characters, but also roles of authorial intent. Taken as a description of a person's identity, it may be difficult to figure out how one reconciles these seemingly disparate roles for the self. In this world of multiple roles, however, identity is made up not only of a profoundly rich ongoing conversation with an external world, but also with a remarkable inner world. The makeup of this ongoing conversation is what the literary critic Mikhail Bakhtin refers to as "dialogical," after the shared, reflective foundation of the life of an individual and the makeup of reality.

The dialogical makeup of a text, which Bakhtin describes with the term "polyphony" (the many-voiced, multiplicitous nature of reality), is one in which elements of a story never exist atomically and in separation from other elements of the story—even the presence of the author—wherein all voices and all things they come to represent maintain worlds unto themselves, all the while reflecting the worlds of every other entity within the story. Although Bakhtin's polyphonic understanding of a text can easily apply to the world one lives in, it just as easily reflects the makeup of a human person's self-identity where "the dialogic nature of consciousness, the dialogic nature of human life itself … exists in the forms *I* and *another*."[7] In much the same fashion, Bakhtin defines the position of an author as a character: "we find the author *outside* the work as a human being living his own biographical life…but we must also meet him as the creator of the work itself, although he is located outside."[8] It is always easy to attempt to construe the relationship between an author and his work, or a person and the immediate world they create for themselves that surrounds them, simplistically, which is to say, by construing the person and their world as being profoundly disentangled or too synonymous. In the dialogical reading of an author's relationship to their work, a vast web of individual entities simultaneously populate a text, reflecting the presence of an author while maintaining a certain amount of autonomy for themselves. Understood as such, it then should not be difficult to transpose Bakhtin's understanding of the function of an author in relation to the characters to how we interpret the multiplicitous nature of both the face and identity. Just as many voices operate and mutually and responsively exist within one text, the same can be said for an individual person. When perceiving in a person's life "an internal connection, *a connection between consciousnesses*,"[9] one should also understand the constitutive makeup of a person to be equally multiple, reflecting the dialogic nature of the world in terms of a complex *internal* dialogue—the same dialogue one finds in an author's relation to his characters as well as to himself. Identity should then be understood as synonymous with the polyphonic position of the author wherein all consciousnesses created within a novel (other characters, plot elements, setting, references, allusions, and even novels outside the novel) are reflected within the consciousness of the author, even when they take on a life of their own.

The celebrity that embodied this principle of self-identity more than any other in the twentieth century, and in fact, a principle he played with as the means to building his reputation, was the controversial comedian Andy Kaufman. Much of Kaufman's strange anticomedy performances consisted of frequently changing roles, transforming appearances while frequently dis-identifying with the name Andy Kaufman (as found with his character, Tony Clifton). When looking at the body of Kaufman's work, even when looking at one of his performances, it is difficult to find a single place where one can point to and say "this is Andy Kaufman." In an "exchange that traversed the craft of his multiplicities in an altogether new manner,"[10] Kaufman, responding to guest host Steve Martin's question about a character he had just played, shows just what Bakhtin had in mind in his description of the position of an author:

A.K.:   What, which one?

S.M.:   The one out there that you did.

A.K.:   Oh, no—that's really me.

S.M.:   Ahhh. And then—

A.K.:   The Foreign Man, you mean? That's another character.

S.M.:   Mmmm-hmmm. So that was really you out there. And then what are you doing right now?

A.K.:   Right now? This is really me.

S.M.:   Oh. [Audience laughter] And then—now, what about the Foreign Man?

AK: No, that's not—that's just a character I do.[11]

Kaufman, a comedic performer of many masks, mimics Bakhtin's understanding of the interaction of characters and author here in an odd way: he treats himself like a polyphonic text. Even when in the interview Kaufman dis-identifies himself with a particular character he plays, he is somehow reflecting and showing the presence of that character's consciousness and the world within his own in much the same way an author does within a novel. By doing so, Kaufman does not identify himself with a single appearance or character, but rather with the *possibility* of a character that he consistently creates in every performance, adding new layers to the name and identity of "Andy Kaufman." The struggle to grow new layers to one's self is the only way to be true and consistent with who one is. Perhaps in this ongoing struggle to renew the covenant with oneself, we find something like a prolonged and transformational version of what Anzieu referred to as the development of a skin ego. When looking at Kaufman's performance, one gains the sense that the growth of a skin ego is never a simple process that reaches a logical conclusion, but is instead a process that is defined through constant regeneration.

In the already crowded scene of the self, making room for new voices is often made difficult by the way people are conditioned to think of identity in terms of one voice. The key to getting beyond this one voice, however, is to hear the micro-tones, the semi-tones, and the varied pitches of this one voice, as well as the influences of others that they indicate. No voice exists in isolation from other voices. This process of reflecting and acknowledging the chorus that makes up one's self also demands a more profound transformation of the plot structure of one's self by always expanding the story of oneself. This is a kind of ongoing understanding of human development that, in the words of the Formalist literary critic

Viktor Shklovsky, "evolves by way of new combinations."[12] By approaching "new combinations" of one's self, the transformation of the human body that results in the creation of what Bakhtin calls a "new bodily canon:"[13] new forms and ways of identifying and representing oneself in the ongoing narrative of one's life. A person must exist with the awareness of the dialogue and story within which their face functions, not merely being one aspect of a person among many, but one aspect with many precisely through creating these combinations of the self. When a person can no longer reflect on how their face interacts with a larger whole and is only cognizant of the face's presence or absence, they can no longer take view of their whole bodies and their whole selves. This experience is something like being trapped within a Bakhtinian bodily canon, where meanings and roles for body parts remain fixed and inflexible. Isn't this the very psychological problem one is often faced with when receiving a face transplant—that one cannot get beyond their face?

The philosopher Gilles Deleuze and the psychoanalyst Felix Guattari were thinking of something similar to Bakhtin's bodily canon when they developed their idea of "faciality" in their sprawling, monumental work *A Thousand Plateaus*. Drawing inspiration from the social function of a face, but not necessarily equating a face with faciality, Deleuze and Guattari outline a way in which a multiplicitous reading of identity can offer means to move beyond the fascinating control one's face can exert over one's entire self-conception. The face, according to Deleuze and Guattari, "is produced only when the head ceases to be a part of the body, when it ceases to be coded by the body, when it ceases to have a multidimensional, polyvocal corporeal code—when the body, head included, has been decoded and has to be overcoded by something we call the face."[14] The face in faciality is an insidious force. It seduces by means of simplicity, the promise of which ultimately proving untrue and resulting in a feeling of immobility. The face in faciality works through overriding attachments that allow a person to see only one aspect of themselves: their face. A person is able to see nothing beyond the face, for the face takes over the whole body, the whole person, severely constraining their possibilities, and the variations of the story that their life might tell. However, if one is able to fight the control that a single face can exert over an entire person's life, one will find the effervescence of growth that the face attempts to thwart. For the sake of engendering this growth, Deleuze and Guattari encourage, "the face has a great future, but only if it is destroyed, dismantled."[15] Moving beyond the constrained "inhumanity of the face,"[16] following what Deleuze and Guattari call "lines of flight," one must generate to a place beyond the face and toward a restored human body of possibilities and variations.

This human body of possibilities is something Deleuze and Guattari describe as a "Body without Organs," a vision of the body where "the question of the body is not one of part-objects but of differential speeds."[17] This body of "differential speeds" is a body much like Bakhtin's dialogical text wherein many autonomous but connected voices underlie all movement and formation of reality. It is the differential speeds, the various stories and narrative possibilities that exist within a person's face, body, and identity that exist as the departure points where "the traits of a face enter a real multiplicity or diagram."[18] When the story of a person—their identity—moves in this direction, the person, their body, and their reality enter a life where they are always assembling and in-process—much like the unfolding of a plot. It is not through some great leap away from a face, radically erasing it leaving a person with a blank head that one achieves the constancy of becoming, but through transforming the facialized head into a head that is capable of sustaining a face that exists dynamically with the rest of the body and that does not result in re-facializing the body.

When a story becomes so fixed in one direction that its plot becomes predictable, the story can no longer progress through surprise or have any real power to communicate or impact the reader. The characters of the story more or less stay locked into the same dialogues, set pieces, and actions with repetitious agony. Allowing a story to progress once again can only be achieved through undermining the undue influence that a particular voice, character, or vision has in limiting the possibility of the story's passage into unknown developments. With the story of the person, this is what Deleuze and Guattari are in some sense aiming to achieve: the total relaxation and reintegration of the dominant voice into the crowd of voices that constitute the existence of any given person. Rather than locating the identity of a person with the facialized mask, Deleuze and Guattari want us to identify the person with their assembled and assembling existence that is always fighting against the smoothing surface of the face. One undoes this smoothing of the face by letting all of the elements of the face rise up, ripple, and create the face's "lines of flight"— the passages from the stagnated face to the face in development.

The gift of a new name, no matter what it is that functions as the designation of one's identity is the trace of movement that connects one's ever multiplying past with the ever developing and emergent future that the *assembling* assemblage is always initiating. The site of facialization then, for Deleuze and Guattari, becomes the point from which shifts, changes, and new aspects of one's self-identity emerge through the organizing influence of the face. Every face contains its own undoing and its own unknown future in which the current face will disappear (think here of the processes of aging and adolescence). As the face forms, so do a variety of characteristics that underlie its constitution, characteristics that can eventually give way to change. Folds, creases, and marks not only designate the contours of the face but point to a future face as "lines of flight," to again use the concept of Deleuze and Guattari. The face draws the body and all of its disparate functions and flows together into the assemblage; it is the connecting emblem whose only existence is found in coordinating the body into a coherent and functioning entity, but it is also that which makes more faces possible. The possibilization of the face is the creation of what Deleuze and Guattari refer to as "content-expression,"[19] an articulation of the fluid *process* and not the static referencing of identity. Part of the connective dimension of the face is that it does not only connect and hold together one's life-world out of social pressure. It is merely the strong over-identifications with a single face that get asserted that result in grave consequences, consequences that Deleuze and Guattari interpret in light of authoritarian control: the restriction of future possibilities.

Now, although Deleuze and Guattari disqualify the actual physical face from being the only implement of facialization, this does not mean that the face does not or cannot serve a facializing function. They elect the face in their concept for good reasons. It is no coincidence that the most expressive part of our bodies is also the place where we often feel most restrained, worried at the consequences of what the sociologist Erving Goffman has referred to as "losing face." All fears that attend to and block expression, however, are merely fears of what might become of a face through visionary expression. So long as fears prevent this genuine entry into the future that is a major component of the temporality of narrative identity, a major aspect of identity will remain neglected. One must see all the times that a face, an identity, and a self come to not only represent and embody, but also hint to by nature of identity's transformative and transitional narrative nature.

In eclipsing the traditional one-to-one correspondence between appearance and inner-self that a representational understanding of identity accords, an understanding of human self-identity as an ever-evolving thoroughly complex entity emerges that not only enlarges our understanding of what we as individuals are, it also opens up new possibilities of what the complex entity of self-identity may come to be. This effort, however, can only be achieved at the expense of narrow understandings of identity and faces that radically simplify the role they play in reality.

FACE TRANSPLANT THERAPY

The first face transplants performed on humans have been remarkable surgical and even aesthetic successes. Not only have surgical teams managed to coach transplanted skin tissue onto the faces of recipients with little trouble through effective immunosuppressant therapy, they have also artfully *translated* the face of one person onto the face of another person. The aesthetic precision employed by surgeons in the world's first face transplants has not only offered a big step up in the appearance and functionality of these people's faces, it has also provided a bridge back to the world from which these people had felt isolated: the world of other humans. Although in no way have the wounds of disfigurement that the various recipients and candidates for face transplants received made them less-than-human, the aesthetic skills of surgeons helped the recipients of the first face transplant procedures have relatively "normal"-looking faces. Doing so has been perhaps less an aesthetic goal as it has been a defense against the stigmatizing gazes of other people. It is these gazes that prevent face transplants from being accepted as a beneficial medical procedure.

Prior to the world's first face transplants, there was something like two fantasies that made the procedure's results seem unlikely success stories. On the one hand, there was something like the fundamental fantasy of a biological incompatibility at work in scientific and popular imaginations. On the other hand, there was something like the fundamental fantasy of a psychological incompatibility that seemed to stem from cultural fantasies of what it meant to both lose one's own face and receive someone else's face in exchange. It was thought too complicated by many to attach the face of one person to that of another. Too many biological facts and medical difficulties stood in the way, genetic qualities and facial bone structure just a few issues among many. The thought that one could ever psychologically cope with or adjust to the transplanted face of another person on one's own head was simply too unfathomable for many, because it seemed to go against every meaning we associate with faces and every conception we give to the idea of identity. Of these two fantasies, one has been put to rest, and one remains spectral.

Developments in composite tissue transplantations—procedures that work with genetically mismatched material—have shown that the requirements of genetic relevance in tissue transplant procedure are, immunologically speaking, fairly if not completely irrelevant. Drugs such as cyclosporine and tacrolimus, as well as careful and skilled medical technique, have proven the great chasm between one and another's DNA to be of little consequence to successful performance of a face transplant. As such, the first fantasy, that of a biological incompatibility, is put to rest. The second fantasy—psychological incompatibility—is not so easily dealt with. One cannot deal with the psychological fears associated with face transplants by coming up with a simple scientific formula; for the psychological problems experienced in receiving a face transplant procedure are as varied and individualized as human faces themselves are, but the solution to this second dilemma is not entirely unrelated to the first.

It has been suggested that certain aesthetic requirements that would seem crucial to psychological adjustment in a face transplant procedure such as race and gender might not be of the slightest importance to candidates for face transplant procedures.[20] Many of these candidates are so eager to obtain the functioning of a face that conventional categories of construing appearance just seem to dissolve when confronted with the biological and psychological alternative of not having a face. Far from fulfilling some sort of twisted eugenicist proposition, the idea that traditional typologies of identity such as race and gender might not be of any real concern in face transplants is an interesting proposition and one that hints at what goes on psychologically within the procedure: the burden of experiencing radical transformations in both personal *and* human identities.

No matter if we describe the recipients of face transplants as visionary or innovative examples of human malleability, each recipient of a face transplant procedure will inevitably have to wrestle with the difficulty of becoming someone different from what they have always known and expected. This challenge of becoming someone unknown for face transplant recipients does not mean that the pressure of moving a species forward in its self-conception falls on the shoulders of their psychological lives—because a duty such as that is far too onerous for any one single person. Without having to also assume the burden that all people share in reimagining what it means to be human, the face transplant recipient must endeavor to reimagine their own identity. Given the way we have offered a reading of identity and faces through the logic of narratives and stories, how might a therapeutic intervention address the psychological task of reimagining identity?

Just as putting the fantasy of a biological incompatibility to rest depended on making people see that it was possible *physically* to receive the face of another person, overcoming the fantasy of a psychological incompatibility between the one person and the face of another entails showing that it is *psychologically* possible to receive the face of another person. Part of this work emerges from the understanding of identity we have just outlined; hints to the other part of this work can be gleaned from what people already do when faced with traumatic moments in their lives. A face means and functions differently for every individual, whether they possess a face or not. The trick to framing any discussion of working therapeutically with the challenging psychological dimension of receiving a face transplant is to be found by showing that receiving a new face and synthesizing it within one's identity is already a familiar practice to the story of one's life.

It could perhaps be argued that there must be a certain level of ego strength present in any prospective recipient of a face transplant without which enduring the identity-shattering experience of receiving someone else's face might be entirely too traumatic. Taking a brief look at recent scholarship on the psychological dimension of face transplant procedures,[21] it is evident that a certain amount of importance has been placed on the role of psychological assessment in determining who is "fit" to receive a face transplant. Although it makes sense to make certain that candidates for this procedure are of a relatively sound psychological state before undergoing a psychologically harrowing procedure, the idea that assessment can ever point to a candidate who will be able to undergo the procedure without a hitch is very naïve. Of course assessing a candidate's psychological coping skills, ego strength, and firm sense of reality are qualities that might make a person more apt to psychologically deal with having the flesh of another person on their body; they are also important for the long-term success of any transplant procedure.

Perhaps commentators who doubted the mental stability of Clint Hallam (the recipient of the world's first hand transplant who later had the hand removed) in retrospect may have a point (however unfair their stigmatization of Hallam's past may be). An overriding emphasis placed on the role of assessment, however, fails to acknowledge the likely response that any person would have to a face transplant or even that only a person with severe body dissociations would ever be able to receive a face transplant with little psychologically traumatic consequence. That being said, there is perhaps something to the importance of assessing the "strength" of one's sense of a life story and how well one weathers difficult transformative moments throughout life. Receiving a new face will feel calamitous to one's sense of identity and will be inevitably experienced to the narrative of one's life, no matter how grave the physical need for a face may be. No matter the positive and promising outcome of any psychological assessment, the idea that one can find a psychologically suitable candidate for the procedure is dubious—at best. The shock one experiences in receiving the face of another person is an experience for which one can have very little preparation. The level to which one's identity is disrupted in a face transplant procedure is rarely experienced throughout life. The trauma of a face transplant is not an experience one can guard against; it is a watershed moment that can only be worked with after the fact. As such, the psychological focus of working with a face transplant recipient must be postdiluvian rather than antediluvian.

By focusing on the psychological life of the face transplant recipient after the procedure, therapists and counselors could help the patient with

the hardest adjustment one must make when identity is traumatically interrupted: synthesizing one's new life with the old.

FACESWAP

In *Playing and Reality*, the British child psychoanalyst D. W. Winnicott
describes an interesting vignette with a patient that is especially salient to
the discussion at hand:

> [T]his same week this patient found a picture of my face on a book cover.
> She wrote to say she needed a bigger version so that she could see the lines
> and all the features of this "ancient landscape." I sent the picture (she lives
> away and I see her only occasionally now) and at the same time I gave her
> an interpretation based on what I am trying to say in this chapter.... This
> patient thought that she was quite simply acquiring the portrait of this man
> who had done so much for her (and I have). But what she needed to be told
> was that my lined face had some features that link for her with the rigidity
> of the faces of her mother and her nurse.... I feel sure that it was important
> that I knew this about the face, and that I could interpret the patient's
> search for a face that could reflect her, and at the same time see that,
> because of the lines, my face in the picture reproduced some of her mother's
> rigidity.[22]

Although Winnicott's story is here primarily meant to illustrate the dialectic of perception and apperception, there is a funny quality to the transition he describes his patient making between the mother's face and his. He
speaks of lines that seem to connect his face to the mother's—those broken
lines of rigidity that tether a person to their past. Even though Winnicott's
patient is searching for a face whose reflection would be comforting and
psychologically nourishing, something keeps drawing the patient to see the
components of her mother's face, a face full of features she finds inad-
equate for her needs. The lines are what are important here. Here, we may
call to mind the Deleuzian "lines of flight" that we spoke of earlier in this
chapter. What Winnicott's patient was in search of was not a face that
could perfectly reflect her own feelings, needs, and emotions; the face she
was in search of was not any particular face but the possibility of developing a new face *within* herself. The task of working with this patient would
no doubt be similar to the task of working with a face transplant recipient.
The course of work that Winnicott would have no doubt pursued with
any client in search of face would have been one of transforming the lines
of rigidity that trammel the future and instead using them as stems from
which the flowers of new growth would flourish. The therapy should not
consist of making an adequate, new face, but allowing the patient to be

freed from the search for the ideal Face and instead be able to create and celebrate ever new faces and facets of their identity.

The term *faceswap,* which seems to have been coined by the surgeon Peter Butler (a man who, as a former artist, perhaps is well suited for appreciating the artistic and literary dimensions of face transplant procedures),[23] proves to be an interesting way of describing the concept that is at play in working therapeutically with recipients of face transplant procedures. Certainly the term applies to Winnicott's vignette wherein, quite literally, his patient is in search of a sort of swapping of faces. Perhaps Butler's term even captures something of the fluidity that keeps the actual medical procedure from being separated from all the psychological work done subsequent to the procedure. Whatever the use or implications of this interesting interdisciplinary term (maybe it should replace "facial allograft" or "face transplant" altogether), the one aspect of working therapeutically with face transplant recipients that the term captures is the necessary merging of elements between the life of a person past and the life of a person to be. Not only does a face transplant procedure create an interesting kind of psychological miscegenation in the life of a person, it even affects an interesting possibility and challenge for the person as a vision of the future, wherein, as a recent article on face transplants put it, "you don't get donor identity transplant, you don't get quite back to where you were ... it's a hybrid."[24]

The hybrid outcome of the procedure, much like the way a film assembles in the editing room, is the fluid movement of identity that must be taken up therapeutically as an emerging narrative process within the patient. Although this is not a story of which a person has total control, charging it with new direction at whim, it is a tale for which a person has ample power in opening up new possibilities and the emergence of new threads. In some sense, a narrative approach to working through the psychological difficulties posed toward one's sense of identity in receiving a new face through a face transplant would work on incorporating one's new face in a process that would both allow a person to relinquish the identity of the past while creating and embracing an identity of the future that is opened up through the perspective of a new face. In some sense, this sort of therapeutic approach would attempt to have one learn to look at one's self *through* their new face and not *at* their new face.

In the case of facial disfigurement, be it as a result of burn injuries, animal attack, or other forms of mutilation, a new face becomes the possibility of a new story for one's life. Joan Didion's famous opening line from *The White Album,* "we tell ourselves stories in order to live,"[25] lends something of a weight and direction to the therapeutic task of working with the psychological fallout of a face transplant. To make the most of one's new face requires a certain sense of how a new face allows a person to live again in a psychical sense. What is so hard about this endeavor? In Chapter 4 we spoke of it in terms of a haunting, an inability to overcome one's powerful identifications with the past that prevent the emergence of a future continuous with the past. Perhaps in something like Dinoire's ambivalent feelings toward her me/not me face we can find a hint at the crisis in narrative that the psychological aspects of face transplants provoke. We have seen how tricky the past has proven in many popular culture representations of transplant procedures, but have also offered the opinion that it is through overcoming and overdetermining the function of one's past that an enlarged sense of possibility for the future and for one's identity emerges. If we are to be able to interpret the development and emergence of face transplant procedures, we must construct a new face for the human being by reconstructing the traditional notion of an "identity" within their life. Much of this work can be done with what people already know about themselves: that they are multifaceted, have immense histories, and have many attachments and interests. So much that makes up a person remains even after the loss of some central emblem of one's identity; rather than viewing all of this as baggage, it might be more helpfully understood as various constitutive lines and flows (in the Deleuzian sense) to one's life, through which one can seek transformation in the most troubling moments of identity crisis. A person is full of elements that the loss of a face may disturb or kick dust upon and with which a new face may seem incompatible. These, however, are the parts of a person for which a new face can offer new perspectives and thus, new life.

In effecting identity, the newly transplanted face can only be incorporated as an element of a new story for a person in so far as the face's impact on every dimension of a person's existence, all of the facets that crisscross the narrative of a person's life, is also examined and considered in the process of incorporating the new face. From pedestrian preferences to more deep seated beliefs, the addition of a new element into a person's world will always cause quite a shake-up. Putting the pieces into place as they fall back from the shake-up is the therapeutic challenge posed by face transplant procedures. In this sense, the psychological treatment of identity issues associated with face transplant procedures is not unlike other sorts of trauma work. As one also finds in psychological work with victims of various sorts of trauma treatment, one can never merely aim to drown out or cover over the traumatic moment or experience. Silencing the unfathomable abyss encountered in such moments skirts the necessary and complicated process of making room within and reordering one's narrative as a result of the traumatic experience. Doing so does not amount to a justification or moral legitimization of what has befallen a person. Instead, one merely endeavors to continue to assemble the story of who they are—of their identity—without having to turn away from traumatic experience. However, as we find with face transplant recipients this kind of assembling process is tricky when working with someone who has lost something that seems so central to their identity.

Working in a narrative fashion with the psychological identity crisis of a face transplant recipient becomes nearly hopeless so long as the therapeutic approach still understands the significance of the face as if it were a mask and the nature of identity as if it were static. Just as the belief that, in a face transplant, one can find a face that will either match a person's identity, properly functioning as a sign for a misunderstood inner world, or perform the procedure in a way that will not jar a patient's self-identity, failing to acknowledge the complex and multifaceted nature of one's identity, will result in a therapeutic process that, at best, will offer short-term cognitive coping skills for the patient who is undergoing a long-term and existential crisis. The up-building of one's "ego" strength in the face of this crisis can only be achieved through the reinforcing and expanding of one's self-identity, not necessarily by adding in ever-new components, but through making a person aware of what already exists within their lives, their past, and their self—in short, adding complexity to one's complexion. The adding on of a new face to one's self, as perplexing and troubling as the experience might be, does not equate to creating a *tabula rasa* out of one's identity. The addition of a new face to the narrative of one's identity is tantamount to adding a new element or figure to one's life, *as well as* a process of moving forward with what already exists to one's identity through a process of reconnecting the heterogeneous pieces of one's life. This reconnecting demands a reconceptualization of the links between some pieces of one's self, how one represents certain aspects of who they are, and connects their personality to themselves without having to start their self over from scratch.

Creating a new story of the self through the perspective of the transplanted face is not achieved by coming up with a new sense-of-self as conjured through a simple story, but through transforming the complex web of processes that make up a person's identity from minute questions of taste to broader questions of social and political roles. Within the story of one's life, a person takes up many different functions, and their personhood and their identity springs forth from the interaction of all of these different roles. Identity somehow coordinates all of this while provoking new connections and new associations within one's life. A person's identity is not a thing, nor is it *simply* a story. To conceive of a person's identity in a narrative fashion, one must understand that the story of a person's life always includes a certain sort of driving force, the energy of a plot that is merely another aspect of our identity. Similar to what Alfred Hitchcock called a "macGuffin," the element within a story around which a plot generates itself, there is an element to one's identity that not only drives forward the story of one's self, it also adds richness, complexity, and opens up new possibilities within the story. Although this driving force interacts with the story, it is something that is also firmly just beyond the grasp of the story, existing as that energy which always seems to open up new directions, paths, and possibilities within a tale. This too is our identity: the parts we have yet to discover.

But identity can trap us to the past just as it can draw us into the future. Any seemingly prosaic element of our world can function as this crucial link. For the recipient of the face transplant procedure, it just so happens to be a face that can both trammel and rejuvenate the narrative. However, the narrative of identity could just as easily hinge on something else, like another body part (echoing the transplant surgeon Dr. John Barker infamous statement, "a face is just like a hand"[26]). Only by moving beyond the all too familiar meanings associated with faces—be they cultural, scientific, or intuitive—can one embrace the more abstract yet highly singular function that a face serves in the life any individual. The truly individualized face, the face that can only ever belong to one person is not made of skin but of possibilities. From this point the road forward from a face transplant begins.

Briefly returning to the three themes that were outlined in this book's introduction—identity, innovative technology, and trauma—any effective approach to the psychological problems that a face transplant procedure stirs forth must not forget the central roles these three themes play when the self faces new and daunting developments for itself. To successfully perform a face transplant, overcoming the biological chasm that exists between genetic mismatches is not enough. For the face to bind itself to recipient and rebind the world of the recipient that was sundered through disfigurement, the face transplant must continue on well after the patient has been wheeled out of the operating room. Yes, the actual medical procedure is a procedure that, in a sense never really ends, as a person must continue to receive continued medical attention as well as a life-long regiment of immunosuppressant drugs. The task of psychologically adjusting in this same fashion does not mean that the trauma of a new face will forever be a haunting experience one will have to endure for all time. The storm of that trauma also recedes as the person grows to adjust to having a new face, reconciling their past to their new face, but the battering winds of that storm are never far from shore when one insists on staying in the same place. Countering our meteorological intuitions, the storm grows less fierce as we travel alongside it; the more we insist on staying in the same spot, the more susceptible we become to a repeated onslaught. When the narrative of identity gets interrupted, one only creates danger by refusing to move in the new direction that interruption takes you.

The storm of uncertainty over the nature of one's identity and existence that is central to the psychological experience of a face transplant is a storm that all humans must face in different ways when they are left asking themselves "who am I?" As cripplingly frightening this question may be for many, it is only by being willing to ask this question that we can ever hope to understand who we are and what we might become. For the face transplant recipient, this hysterical question offers the possibility of piecing one's world back together by first acknowledging that it has come apart. When one's identity falls apart, one must put it back together through the story that the new face offers—a story that is waiting to be told, but before the story can move forward, one must resolve to not fear the traumatic shock of the new—a shock that, in giving a new a face to one, gives a new face to all.

Conclusion

Simon Weston, a well-known veteran of Britain's Falklands War of the early 1980s, is the patron of one of the most forward-thinking organizations that is working toward the performance and dissemination of face transplant procedures, Dr. Peter Butler's The Face Trust. While serving in the British Army during the Falklands War, the British Fleet ship on which Weston was serving was bombed by enemy planes, exploding fuel supplies and ammunition aboard ship, covering half of Weston's body with severe burn injuries including areas of his face. In the years since the Falklands War, Weston has undergone dozens of reconstructive surgeries for burned areas on his face, becoming a celebrity of sorts in the United Kingdom through various charitable commitments. As Weston has been somewhat of a success story for recipients of facial reconstructive surgeries, his involvement with advocating for face transplant procedures has been intriguing. Although Weston himself has expressed no interest in being the recipient of the procedure, he stands as one of the more outspoken public figures for the procedure in the United Kingdom today. Butler, the surgeon who heads up The Face Trust, has considered performing a face transplant on a number of people, including veterans of current armed conflicts in the Middle East. Not only are wounded and disfigured war veterans now considered as potential candidates for face transplants, Butler has gone on the record saying that he would give priority to treating a wounded war veteran, telling *The Times*, "we definitely would offer treatment to any veterans who approached us.... We owe a debt to these people."[1] Weston himself agrees with Butler, seeing a clear need to perform the procedure for many who have been disfigured by combat injuries. Speaking to *The Times*, Weston has said that, "there may be soldiers who have been disfigured for the past four years who may feel that they are so unhappy with their appearance they may wish to look at different alternatives.... Face transplant is the only option for full reconstruction."[2]

Although no face transplants have been performed on any war veterans from Iraq or Afghanistan as of yet, the possibility of using a face transplant for many wounded and disfigured veterans is an interesting proposition. Shortly after news of the face transplant performed at the Cleveland Clinic broke to the media, the transplant team, led by Maria Siemionow, announced that it had received a grant from the U.S. Department of Defense to explore the use of face transplant procedures on war verterans at an army medical center in Texas.[3] With the procedure having been performed only a few times since its first successful completion in 2005, the future of faces transplants is still largely undetermined. To a certain extent, there isn't even a guarantee that face transplants will not be written off at some point in time in the future as a fluke of modern medicine, having failed ever to gain wide-scale acceptance in culture and in the medical community (although many doctors voice their support for the procedure). Part of what threatens the future of face transplants, as well as what makes the procedure still very exciting, is its lack of direction in application. For whom will the procedure proliferate? Thus far the procedure has been performed on victims of animal attacks and on a man whose face was so laden with tumors that his speaking and eating was significantly impaired. Although from these procedures one can get a sense of the possibilities and range of the procedure, one can hardly extrapolate a clear program for implementing the procedure from the first three cases of face transplants. It has been suggested that face transplants might be an important palliative solution for burn victims.[4] As with the third recipient of a face transplant, who suffered from the genetic disease neurofibromatosis, surgeons might ponder the possibilities of focusing the procedure on those with certain genetic conditions that severely affect their appearance, as well as the function of their face. All are interesting cases, but there is something compelling about the idea of using face transplant procedures with war veterans.

Anyone who needs a face transplant procedure is likely to have severe psychological problems and identity issues associated with a condition that would necessitate such a surgical intervention. Given the fact that disfigured war veterans already face high stakes in their struggle for psychological well-being as a result of their disfigurement (the position in which anyone in need of a face transplant finds themself), they may very well be likely candidates for the procedure. With at least 300 American soldiers having suffered injuries of significant facial disfigurement while in combat, the immediate demand for the use of face transplant procedures for war veterans should be clear enough. Yes, soldiers in past wars have also faced the dangers of facial injuries, but the nature of war in current conflicts— often guerrilla in nature, such as the frequent threat of roadside bombs— exposes soldiers to even greater threats of facial injuries and more severe facial wounds sustained than in either World War I or World War II.[5] With reconstructive surgeries already being performed on soldiers coming back from war with facial wounds[6]—burns, collapsed noses, and lost portions of face structure among other injuries—face transplants would seem to be the next logical step in treating soldiers with facial injuries.

An even more compelling argument for the use of face transplant procedures with wounded veterans stems from the psychology of trauma experiences in war. Following the idea that we developed in the last chapter of the narrative nature of identity that face transplants help to underscore, it is perhaps helpful to point out that the trauma experienced by soldiers in war, be it physical in nature or not, is often the problem of the loss of one's sense of self—the shattering of one's identity—through the disruption of their identity. Not only have many soldiers been badly disfigured while serving during recent armed conflicts in the Middle East, but the traumatic impact of war and the associated way that it has been a disruptive presence in the life of wounded soldiers is another hidden dimension of injury that each physically wounded soldier bears after the wartime experience. The experience of a disfiguring war wound is a rather complex problem for a soldier. Such a complex problem demands a complex solution; face transplant procedures might just be that solution. By offering face transplant procedures to veterans, one not only distinguishes the role of face transplants for disfigured veterans as individuals and as a group, one also identifies the important role that face transplant procedures might serve for a nation. In some ways, the nation itself has been wounded by the most recent armed conflicts for different reasons—losing a family member or friend, feeling lied to about the nature of the way Iraq War has played out, and soldiers' feeling betrayed by their fellow citizens (in a variety of different ways), among others. Although performing face transplant procedures on certain wounded and disfigured soldiers would not solve all of these problems, it might offer the opportunity to transform much of the pain experienced in the Iraqi and Afghan conflicts into something defined less by the strictures of pain and more by the possibility of hope.

And yet, the usefulness of face transplants is not necessarily clear to all people. A recent high-profile article from a major newspaper highlighted the problem of facial injuries with American war veterans and made no mention at all of face transplants, in spite of mentioning other options.[7] Face transplants themselves are no real newcomers to war. Although the technology to perform transplants was not around during World War I, the British had a specialized army corps called the "Masks for Facial Disfigurement Department."[8] Situated in the 3rd London General Hospital and jokingly referred to as "The Tin Noses Shop,"[9] the Masks Department was in charge of sculpting and creating an assortment of facial prostheses—more or less masks—that would mimic as closely as possible the way a wounded soldier's face looked before their injury. Although the results could, at times, be masterful, the mask was just simply not a face, and it would take decades before the promise of reconstructive techniques would be refined and safe enough for regular use on facial injuries.

With stories such as that of "The Tin Noses Shop," one can appreciate how much the face has been distinguished in its vulnerability in the history of war. If one were to go through *The Iliad*, for instance, and note every gruesome injury and death that result, your book would soon be left ragged and dog-eared. Even though disfigurement as a result of injuries in war can come in a variety of forms, the danger for the face in war is often greater, for the risks in having it injured are higher. The face in danger during the time of war is not simply the physical face through which people identify one another; the face in danger is the face of identity; in every war injury and experience of trauma stands a great risk posed to the security one feels in relation to the sense of self.

The shattering experience of having one's life thrown into turmoil by an injury, or by the simple experience of having been in combat can often be enough to leave a soldier disillusioned and troubled by what his eyes have seen; it is often enough to bring down the world around that person. The risks of war far exceed the risks of everyday life, and as such, identity occupies a much more precarious place for a solider when at war.

Technology has something do with this whole picture of the fragility of the face in war. One of the major themes on which the German Expressionist art movement focused was the ravages to life caused by the First World War. Many of the artists involved with the movement, as citizens of Central Europe and frequently as soldiers, experienced many of these sorts of atrocities firsthand, including the wide-scale problem of disfigurement that was unleashed by the technology of modern warfare. The use of new weapons made to be more violent and to function with greater scope, more speed, and an enlarged range of distance exposed many soldiers to a level of shock and precariousness unprecedented in the history of ancient and modern warfare.[10]

For the Expressionist painter Otto Dix, the questions of war, disfigurement, and technology were of a special interest, as one sees in what is perhaps his most famous painting, *Der Skatspieler* (The Skat Players; 1920). Dix's painting portrays the experience of combat injury in as vivid a picture of disfiguration than can perhaps be found anywhere else in visual portrayals of war and its effects. The painting portrays three figures, each a war veteran, ensconced around a table playing a game of cards. Each player somehow does not appear as he should, with each veteran a mangled mix of disfigured and improbably positioned limbs, exposed and wounded human body parts intertwined with the workings of machine parts that guide the movements of each player around the table. With a room illuminated by a grim, *memento mori* light bulb, we see a veteran holding his cards with his foot, the leg angled up like an arm with a face whose mouth has slid to one side, missing an eye, and without an ear; in its place runs a long metallic ribbed tube connected to a horn on the table with which he listens to his fellow card players. At first glance, it is difficult to glean what the subject of Dix's painting is. Painted in a grotesque style (later denounced as "degenerate" by Nazis), Dix's painting seems to present the very conundrum in which the wounded and traumatized of today's armed conflicts in the Middle East stand—a crossroads of the old, the new, technology, and the self—an intersection that is confirmed by empirical research today.[11, 12]

Just as greater risks posed by technologically advanced weapons opened up a greater vulnerability for soldiers' identities and bodies in wars past, soldiers today face similar, yet historically unforeseen risks when involved in the waging of war. The trauma of war, although not new or unique to current armed conflicts, takes on new problems and new question(s) in each war, but one problem every soldier faces, no matter what war one is speaking of, is the long and, in some ways, occluded journey back to their homes away from war.

The psychiatrist Jonathan Shay attempts to examine this very problem of the soldier's harrowing excursion home from war through the prototypical and mythological version of this exact journey: the Homeric warrior Odysseus's quest to find his way back to Greece after the fall of Troy. Shay's work, *Odysseus In America*, is an attempt to interpret more contemporary problems of war trauma—the experience of posttraumatic stress disorder (PTSD) and grave feelings of distrust that veterans feel toward the world around them—through a reading of Homer as commentator on the struggles of the soldier as hero.[13]

Also an author of a well-known book that looks at war trauma and Vietnam veterans through the scope of more Ancient Greek mythology,[14] Shay attempts to document and discuss the problems traumatized soldiers face in their bid to return to the worlds they have left behind when they

went off to war. Seeing the struggles of war veterans as unfortunate episodes in the evolution of an endless (and unnecessary) tragedy, Shay's book
offers an interesting idea: what keeps soldiers from returning home is an
inability to start a new story in the moral struggle to regain a grip on their
life after war. Following Shay's use of Homer's *Odyssey* as a metaphor for
the soldier's experience, it is also possible to understand the experience of
disfigurement as a form of trauma within the story of a person's life: a
stumbling block on the road home from war.

Richard Kelly's postapocalyptic film *Southland Tales*, although a monumental critical and commercial flop, presented a sci-fi Los Angeles placed
under martial law and was narrated by a disfigured Iraq War veteran
played by the musician Justin Timberlake. The film, depicting a world
wrought by the aftereffects of nuclear bomb attack, was the first film
released by a major film studio to feature a disfigured Iraq War veteran.
Although the film does not do much in terms of elaborating on Timberlake's character's experience of disfigurement, it is interesting to observe it
in the context of a world turned upside down. Similar to something such
as Cormac McCarthy's novel, *The Road*, an equally terrifying depiction of
the world experienced *after* time, the question of how one returns to a
world after it has been destroyed, as we find in Kelly's film, raises issues
not only of feeling alienated from a world where one doesn't belong, and
the obvious elements of identity to such a feeling, but that the experience
of a loss of identity as a war veteran stems from the feeling that time has
run out, that the world no longer exists, and that there is no longer a map
with which one can make sense of their life. The direction to the narrative
of one's life has disappeared, and in its place rests a complicated and troubling question.

When the road back has fallen into disrepair, how does one find the
way home? One difficulty that Shay fails to point out in his otherwise
compelling examination of war trauma is that traumatized soldiers—and
for our purposes here, the disfigured soldier—inevitably find themselves
somehow trapped outside of the experience of time, a scenario where soldiers, having had the story of their lives disrupted, are no longer capable of
experiencing a narrative of promise and future. Instead, what injured veterans of war encounter is the endless odyssey of the consequences of trauma:
a journey that can feel to be without end or relief.

In the book *Purple Hearts: Back from Iraq*, photographer Nina Berman
compiled a number of interviews she conducted with Iraq War veterans
whom she was photographing, veterans who had all experienced some sort
of wartime injury with resultant physical trauma. Berman's book contains
an array of stories and narratives, told by soldiers, that serve as companion

pieces for documentary photographs of soldiers, young, old, male, and female, who share their life stories of existing with various types of war wounds, disfigurements, and trauma, such as brain damage, facial disfigurement, loss of limbs, and paralysis. Each story presents a different experience, each unique within the context of the book. In one interview, a twenty-one-year-old man who lost sight in both of his eyes and lost one of his legs stated with pride: "I don't have any regrets. No not at all. It was the best experience of my life."[15] Here, speaking to the negative sentiment that this same soldier had perceived in declamations against the war: "one of the biggest things that's wrong with people nowadays, they're so anti-military. Not in the sense where they don't want a military, but they don't want our military involved in a conflict. And that's what makes us America."[16] Strongly patriotic words. Being a veteran, this man's sense of patriotism might be taken for granted; however, his sentiment is still somewhat surprising, given the fact that he not only lost a leg, but also the use of his sense of sight. However, what appears at first to be a contradictory aspect of a man's experience from one perspective, is really a glimpse of the immense scope of the experience of war, as well as an example of the complex levels that exist in a veteran's sense of identity after war.

Another story from Berman's book reads, "yeah, I got a Purple Heart. I don't care. No soldier wants a Purple Heart. I'll tell you that much. No soldier wants it. Awards don't mean nothing to me. I don't need anything to prove I was there. I know I was there. I got a constant reminder."[17] The reminders of war, the physical presence of one's traumatic experiences in combat not only seem to bind people to their experiences, they even occlude the possibilities of the future. Another soldier who Berman interviews perhaps best describes the internal wanderings of the traumatized soldier better than any myth could: "here I am, back here. I would love to go away. I would love to go away. I think that would be better. Because I'm driving in my car, I'm doing nothing. I don't know where it's going to end up."[18] By simply allowing soldiers the opportunity to openly express their feelings about their experiences in war, Berman makes the powerful therapeutic move of making room for individual stories within larger collective narratives of the war experience—a process that enables veterans to see how the war has impacted them individually instead of as a whole. Not only does Berman's work begin to give voice to the difficulties these war veterans have faced and are facing, her work clues a nation in on the problems they face through the collaborative creation of what a reviewer of Berman's work referred to as "tip-of-the-iceberg images."[19] The images that Berman coconstructs with the veterans she photographs begin to hint at the immense problems of trauma, disfigurement, and identity that exist under the surface of all war experience.

As soldiers take harrowing steps back from war to home, what is most needed for them is to be embraced by the place to which the are returning in a way that allows them to be released from the bonds of shame, pride, and guilt that prevent them from moving forward with their lives. As is stated in the introduction to Berman's book, "no one has the right to say that these soldiers are not heroes.... To a soldier coming home from war, the word "hero" looks surprisingly like a gesture of incomprehension, especially in our time when the word is on everyone's lips."[20] Trauma hollows people out; understanding this trauma and the effects that it has on people's sense of self and identity is the first crucial step to be taken in moving on. How, then, have the military, the medical, and the psychiatric communities responded to this abyss of trauma that Berman's photos and interviews only hint at? How have they answered the need to aid the healing, storytelling process of a war veteran's road home?

In an army report of 2005, already more than 1,000 troops had reported symptoms of PTSD[21]; even with little doubt that the number has grown considerably in the years since, the Department of Defense reports that soldiers are less likely to seek out traditional mental health services in cases of PTSD due to the stigma that many in the military attach to psychological problems.[22] With many soldiers avoiding any sort of psychological treatment of counseling of their problems with war trauma due to a stigmatized understanding of mental "illness," the question of responding to the problem of war trauma has become trickier for the branches of the United States military. As an increasing number of soldiers that come back from war are unable to adjust to life away from wartime, the army has had to conjure new forms of treating the physical and psychological problems of war. In response to mounting cases of war trauma and PTSD, the U.S. Army, Navy, and Marines have developed and implemented programs of stress management aimed at preparing for the situations that provoke PTSD symptoms as well controlling its outbreak while at war. In both the Army's CSC (Combat Stress Control) and the Navy/Marines' OSCAR (Operational Stress Control And Readiness), psychological service providers are included as peers in overseas military operations, serving as counselors and mental health educators with soldiers at war.[23] The idea behind programs such as OSCAR is that, by having embedded psychological service providers existing alongside soldiers serving in combat, soldiers might be able to more immediately address ongoing problems of traumatic experiences in war. Although stress control and readiness in a time of war seems somewhat contradictory, the approach at least acknowledges the need to help soldiers process the experience of war. However, operational stress and the larger problems experienced as wellsprings of war trauma often factor in the experience of war at different levels of scale. Soldiers will always find ways to diffuse the tension of serving in combat through the various methods that they always have; as such, the presence of counselors, intending to forestall the more painful experiences of war, will only serve the slightest consolatory roles in the most difficult of experiences. The idea of obviating trauma in a time of war is something like a psychological pipe dream: it will never be successful.[24] Programs such as OSCAR, even if relatively progressive in their approach to trauma, show that the response to trauma by the military, as well as medical and psychological professionals on the whole, has been somewhat underwhelming.

For instance, in the array of treatments that have emerged for PTSD—eye desensitization therapy, various cognitive-behavior treatments, and pharmaceuticals—most aim at the quick containment, control, and normalization of symptoms of PTSD, leading soldiers away from meaningful discussions of their traumatic experiences in some way, only aiming for the reduction of symptoms of PTSD. The problems of treating the consequences of traumatic experiences in this manner can best be understood by taking a look at what has been considered the most innovative and vanguard of all treatments used with veterans of current armed conflicts: virtual reality therapy.

Initially developed as a graded exposure treatment for people with a crippling fear of heights,[25] virtual reality therapy has come to be used for people suffering from other fears, such arachnophobia, but has gained most acceptance and use in treating victims of mass trauma, from Balkan refugees to victims of 9/11. The method of virtual reality therapy (or, alternatively, virtual reality cognitive flooding or virtual reality imaginal exposure therapy) is simple enough in its application: rig a person up to a machine and have them relive traumatic events. The patients in the therapy sessions wear LCD (liquid crystal display) goggles and are attached to various other modules that recreate the affective dimension of an experience, allowing "for the gradual introduction and control of "trigger" stimuli in the VE in real time that is required to foster the anxiety modulation needed for therapeutic habituation."[26] The idea behind virtual reality therapy is that recipients, through repeated exposure to stressors in a virtual environment, will eventually experience a lowering of symptoms. Although studies have shown a decline in the symptoms manifested by sufferers of PTSD,[27] the results are perhaps insidious; results obtained through making a person repeatedly experience the source of a painful and disturbing moment from their life seem suspicious.

The simple truth of virtual reality therapy is that it functions by distracting people from the pain of their symptoms,[28] which is to say it leads them away from the particular story in which the trauma has served as a moment of interruption. Michael Kramer, a clinical psychologist at the Veterans Administration hospital in Manhattan has said, regarding the use of virtual reality therapy, "we can put them back in the moment;"[29] many find this feature of virtual reality treatment to be virtuous, which seems odd. For instance, there is the obvious question: why on earth would you want to return someone to such a moment? Certainly, to overcome difficult experiences of the past, one must be willing to "return" to them in some sense, but not to lose sight of them, nor to lose the qualities of the experience, but simply to draw new associations with the past. This is a fairly common sense way of approaching painful memory. However, this is not the sort of "return to the moment" that virtual reality therapy technicians have in mind; in place of new associations with the past, virtual reality therapy asks a participant to endure the very conditions in which one first experienced trauma—a warped sort of time travel. For some researchers, simply recreating the visual experience in revisiting trauma is not enough. Psychologist Skip Rizzo, a proponent of virtual reality therapy, even believes that one day, "the therapy will include other stimuli, such as vibrations to stimulate the impact of bombs or rumbling of tanks, and even the smells of war—the body odor, garbage and spices of urban combat, for example."[30] What one encounters as a result is not the meaning of one's trauma, but only the affect. Affect without context can hardly serve any therapeutic function, for it is only the raw sensory information of experience, deprived of the world in which it was first encountered.

Although circumventing the "stigma"[31] of the therapy process that keeps so many soldiers from addressing their difficulties with war trauma, repeatedly immersing recipients in the vortex of their painful memories in a purely sensory way, habituating them to those painful memories, completely avoids the *experience* of having experienced trauma, which is to say, the unique way that a soldier has *narrated* their trauma. Rather than making sense of what has happened to a person, revisiting the experience of trauma, retaining the events but readdressing them as to allow them to affect a person in a new way, merely seeks to erase the trauma, normalizing the experience, by robbing the recipient of the truth of their traumatic experience, creating not only a moral justification for the individual's experience of trauma and war, but also an ontological justification for it: where there is no pain, there can be no sense of injustice or having had something terrible befall one's life. Although these are not sentiments to which one should cling *in perpetua*, it seems as though there is a better way of forming new associations to the past than erasing the feelings of the past. The habituation of one's painful symptoms not only misinterprets the presence of the symptoms of PTSD, normalizing symptoms silences the uniqueness of the traumatized person's experience in negating the presence of affect needed by memory to offer a sense of hope found in the possibility of future experience. In light of the problem of the soldier without narrative, trapped outside of time, therapeutic methods such as virtual reality therapy[32] not only do not give them the healing experience of resuming the flow of time in their lives, this sort of treatment normalizes the time and narrative of war in their lives, effectively keeping the soldier at war— being trapped in the affective time of war means being at war all of the time. Where is the promise of hope for a new story to be found in this?

Face transplants offer hopeful solutions to the complex psychological and physiological problem of disfiguration suffered in facial injuries in war. However, there are certain lessons that must be gleaned from the ways that other emergent forms of technology have failed in their attempted treatment of the psychological problems that result from serving in war. As such, it is quite possible that face transplant procedures may get taken up as virtual reality therapy has, with the best of intentions, but with the poorest of planning and conceptualization of use. With new problems of trauma, as well as the stigma attached to traditional forms of psychological treatment demanding a new therapeutic vision for treatment of trauma symptoms, the stakes are higher for a responsible and well thought out implementation of emerging treatment techniques with veterans of war. What is often overlooked in the advent of new approaches to old problems such as virtual reality treatment of PTSD is the way that seemingly innovative approaches to problems can often blind people with newness to their inadequacies in application. With so many worries permeating our society over the quality of care given to injured veterans, new treatment technology demands closer philosophical examination of its intended use and consequences before it is unleashed on any individual.

What the leading array of PTSD treatments fails to touch on is how trauma impacts one's identity, how it sunders the flow of experience and time in one's life, leaving the traumatized person stuck in a situation without hope. The purpose of treating war trauma is not merely to influence the presence of symptoms and psychological pain, to only reduce the presence of anxiety in fear in everyday life; more paramount is the need to allow veterans, and anyone else traumatized by war, the opportunity to experience life differently, not having negated the influence of trauma on a person's life, but having transformed it into something else. One can only transform the pain of trauma by rearticulating what trauma has deprived the person of: a connection to a world around them.

Giving the wounded soul their due in a way that does not deprive them of their subjective experience of war allows them to transform the pain of loss, shock, and trauma into a hopeful future arrived at through under-standing and treating problems of war trauma in a narrative fashion. We have seen hints of this sort of approach above in our description of the photography of Nina Berman, as well as the interviews she conducts with soldiers she photographs, but taking pictures and interviewing soldiers, although incredibly palliative, is no anodyne solution. Where Berman's work leaves off, in the way it only hints at the larger problems associated with serving recent armed conflict in the Middle East, more holistic, proc-ess focused, and creative approaches to the problems of war trauma might pick up. Following the thread of a wounded, disfigured, or psychologically traumatized soldier and allowing the soldier the opportunity to lead him-self or herself toward a narration of their experience of war, would open up new possibilities for their life. Work of this sort is necessarily interdisci-plinary. Attempted approaches at treating war trauma such as the develop-ment of virtual reality therapy through the collaboration of psychologists and videogame designers could hardly be called "interdisciplinary" in the sense that we have in mind. Attempts such as those found in virtual reality therapy fail to meet and tackle the problem of the disruption of one's iden-tity with the necessary complexity and theoretical and cultural richness that such a problem warrants. Although the use of virtual reality treatment is laudable for the way it attempts to respond to the problem of the stigma with which military personnel often regard traditional psychological treat-ment, its implementation has thus far largely ignored the crucial dimen-sion of an *individual's experience* with war trauma by glossing over the way in which individual experience is impacted by war by focusing only on the pain and symptoms of war trauma—mere markers of deeper psychological disruptions. Because the current use of virtual reality therapy reifies a symptomatic understanding of trauma rather than an understanding that regards trauma as the disruption of the personal narrative of one's life, it will never capture and work with the full scope of individual identity and the experience of war.

Even though face transplants offer immense hope for soldiers who have experienced severe facial disfiguration, the procedure itself is not enough to address the complexity of trauma experienced in war-related injury. Responding to a problem as complex as war trauma, be it physical or psy-chological, demands a unique interdisciplinary collaboration among experts from various fields of study, including those falling outside of the realm of the natural sciences. By expanding what one means by a face transplant procedure in an interdisciplinary fashion, face transplants might very well transform into the ideal way of treating soldiers who have been impacted by profound disfiguration. From the get-go, face transplants already rely

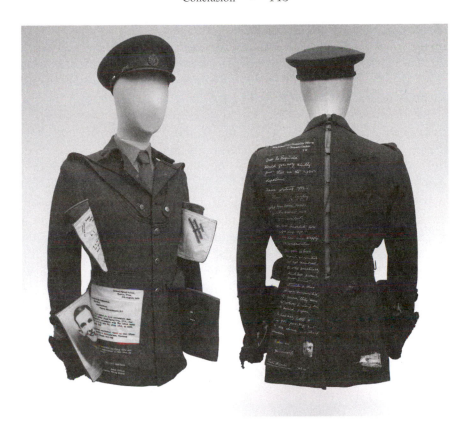

"Lumley," from Paddy Hartley, Project Façade. 2008. Media: Officer's uniform, digital embroidery, appliqué. "Lumley" is in the permanent collection of the Museum of Arts & Design, New York. Image courtesy of artist Paddy Hartley

on an interdisciplinary medical approach including dermatological, epidemiological, and cosmetic concerns that implies an expanded focus in "treating" a patient through the procedure.

An example of this sort of unique interdisciplinarity can be found in the British art project, Project Façade, undertaken by the artist Paddy Hartley. Drawing from old file photos, descriptions of war wounds, war experiences, and the material culture of the First World War, Hartley attempts to creatively reimagine the experiences of disfigured and wounded soldiers of the First World War through the creation of art exhibits that feature expressionistic use of soldiers' dress from the First World War, masks, images, and medical knowledge—sort of like a "Tin Noses" shop for art galleries. Drawing on art, military history, art history, medicine, and mechanical engineering, Hartley takes the traumatic experience of wartime injury out of its the past, rereading and recontextualizing the experience of war injury on a global scale, offering the opportunity to examine the traumatic experience of war, injury, and disfigurement from a place of possibility rather than the constraints of the past.

Might not a unique approach to the problem of the memory of war not serve as a model for how face transplants, as a therapeutic process, might be conceived in the future? A highly interdisciplinary approach, such as is found in Project Façade, could serve as an inspiration for how one might begin to rethink what it means to perform a face transplant procedure. This would impact not only the structure of treatment attached to the surgical procedure, but also the purpose and direction of the process of "healing" in the event of a face transplant. Situating the procedure within the context of a narrative healing is the only hope of addressing the unpredictable problems of identity that any face transplant procedure will provoke. Face transplant procedures may offer such an opportunity to disfigured veterans suffering from the psychological crisis of war trauma by enabling them to find a way to overcome the sundering of one's identity by offering them both a new face and an open possibility of exploring their life story in new ways. There is likely to be a great and unpredictable value for face transplant surgeons, psychiatrists, Department of Defense personnel, and any other individuals taking up the question of a person's life story/identity in a fashion similar to what one finds with the collaborative art/cultural memory found in Hartley's Project Façade; by simply listening to and working with stories of individual soldiers, as found in Nina Berman's work; and by examining the profound cultural, political, and social milieus that soldiers occupy through creative, therapeutic means, as one finds in the work of Otto Dix.

Suggesting an interdisciplinary approach in designing a face transplant process in this way even asks if having consulting writers, artists, art historians, and other academic scholars from the humanities might not benefit from the conceptualization of a face transplant case. Not only could such a team develop a unique and interesting way of approaching and planning the procedure, they would be able to coordinate a highly inventive and appropriately complex healing process that comes after the face transplant. A suggestion such as this need not be considered wishful thinking or unrealistic, for the presence of experts in the craft of narratives such as writers and literary scholars, could offer an immensely helpful contribution to maneuvering a procedure that effects one's identity as much as a face transplant does. The therapeutic process of giving someone a face transplant, as we have already established, does not end with the procedure. The more this insight is incorporated into the healing process of receiving a face transplant, the less likely the psychological problem of identity will occur as greatly as it has otherwise. Working with the face in such an interdisciplinary, complex, and narrative way is not only an innovative way of taking up face transplant procedures, it also models a unique and novel way of tackling the problems of trauma and identity in general.

Here broaching the question of the ethics of face transplants in light of the problem trauma and disfigurement in war veterans raises an interesting question: how does one begin to articulate ethical guiding principles for the use of face transplants?

When technology alone is not enough to save one from the grips of trauma, people must aid technology with the most outstanding skill that humans possess: storytelling. Only by taking up technological interventions, such as face transplants, in a narrative fashion can problems as profound as trauma and identity be fully addressed. Without a guided process of implementing use of face transplants in this sort of narrative manner, the risks and dangers of the technology will always outweigh its benefits. A face transplant will only be helpful for its recipient in so far as it offers the possibility of enriching the narrative of one's life through putting a new face to one's identity. But this story must be the story of the recipient, of the identity for which the face is giving a voice and hope. The new story cannot be the story of the surgeons, the hospital, the military, or anyone else; it is a story that will include all such characters, but the face's future must be created for the immediate benefit of the recipient of the face transplant alone. In aiding the narrative process of overcoming the loss of one's face, one must make sure that the face the person receives is theirs to become and not the face of another person's identity. Although fantasies of the transplanted face's former existence will inevitably start to creep into the psyche of the recipient, the recipient must have the sense that their new face is, in fact, their own—not a negation of their old face, but a transformation of who they are.

To protect against the misuse of an innovative medical procedure such as a face transplant, people must resist turning away from the future that the face transplant procedure has opened up. Mythologies, legends, and stories about emergent phenomena within culture must not evade the inevitable problem of trauma, innovative technology, and identity. Whenever one of these problems arises, the other two are implied, framing the experience as a situation to which one must give a new face. The shock of the new—the fear, anxiety, and self-doubt it creates—can only be addressed by yielding to the possibility that a new face be given to the situation, allaying fear and doubt, while opening up new possibilities for hope, growth, and progress through the transformation of what had so hatefully initially appeared in one's life. Without this, the face of promise and hope, a person will remain in grief and pain, forever reliving the trauma that deprived the person of their face and their identity. Ultimately, the founding principle of an ethical approach to new procedures and the treatment of unprecedented injury should extend from the idea that healing will only come once the process of storytelling has begun to flourish again in one's life. A new face will help to tell the tale; be it physical or not, the story-telling principles that a face embodies will not only lead people toward understanding and away from fear, but it will help guide us through the next trauma, the next innovation, and the next chapter of ourselves.

Notes

INTRODUCTION

1. Liz Kowalczyk, "Brigham Doctors Will Do Rare Face Transplants," *The Boston Globe,* July 29, 2007.

2. Ibid.

3. Dan Glaister, "US Doctors Prepare for First Human Face Transplant," *The Guardian*, September 19, 2005, http://www.guardian.co.uk/world/2005/sep/19/health.usa.

4. Jo Revill, "First UK Face Transplant is in Jeopardy" *The Observer*, July 8, 2007, http://www.guardian.co.uk/society/2007/jul/08/health.medicineandhealth.

5. Bill Hewitt, "Face Transplant Update: It Will Never Be Me," *People*, July 23, 2007, 108.

6. Renshaw et al., "Informed Consent for Facial Transplantation," *Transplant International* (2006): 861–67.

7. G. J. Agich et al., "Until They Have Faces: The Ethics of Facial Allograft Transplantation," *Journal of Medical Ethics* (2005): 707–9.

8. Jon Bowen, "Gaining Face," Salon.com, May 19, 1999. http://www.salon.com/health/feature/1999/05/19/face_transplants.

9. Craig S. Smith, "As A Face Transplant Heals, Flurries of Questions Arise," *The New York Times*, December 14, 2005, http://www.nytimes.com/2005/12/14/science/14face.

10. Wendy Doniger, "Transplanting Myths of Organ Transplants," in *Organ Transplantation: Meanings and Realities*, ed. S. J. Youngner, R. C. Fox, and L. J. O'Connell (Madison, WI: University of Wisconsin Press), 195.

11. We will later see that the Frankenstein myth even served as source material for a B-movie adaptation of it in the 1960s, but it is an adaptation that hits even more close to home for face transplant procedures.

12. Sigmund Freud, *Dora: An Analysis of a Case of Hysteria* (1905; New York: Touchstone, Simon & Schuster, 1997).

13. Ibid., vii–viii.

14. Ibid., 215.

15. Ceclia Hall, "Full-face Transplant Gets Go-ahead," *Telegraph*, October 27, 2006, http://www.telegraph.co.uk/news/uknews/1532394/Full-face-transplant-gets-go-ahead.

CHAPTER 1

1. David Hafetz, "Chasing Hope," *Austin American-Statesman*, May 12, 2002.

2. David Hafetz, "A Face Adds Power to Anti-DWI Effort," *Austin American-Statesman*, October 4, 2002.

3. Roger Highfield and Hall, Celia, "First British Face Transplant 'Within a Year,'" *The Telegraph*, December 20, 2005, http://www.telegraph.co.uk/news/uknews/1505905/First-British-face-transplant-'within-a-year'.

4. Orit Brawer Ben-David, *Organ Donation and Transplantation: Body Organs as an Exchangeable Socio Cultural Resource* (Westport, CT: Praeger, 2005), 46–47.

5. Some examples of these books are, among others: Lesley A. A. Sharp, *Strange Harvest: Organ Transplants, Denatured Bodies, and the Transformed Self* (Berkeley, CA: University of California Press, 2006); Nikolas Rose, *The Politics of Life Itself: Bio-Medicine, Power, and Subjectivity in the Twenty-First Century* (Princeton, NJ: Princeton University Press, 2006); Orit Brawer Ben-David, *Organ Donation and Transplantation: Body Organs as an Exchangeable Socio-Cultural Resource*; Nicholas L. Tilney, *Transplant: From Myth to Reality* (New Haven, CT: Yale University Press, 2003); Michelle Goodwin, *Black Markets: The Supply and Demand of Body Parts* (New York: Cambridge University Press, 2006); Margaret Lock, *Twice Dead: Organ Transplants and the Reinvention of Death* (Berkeley, CA: University of California Press, 2001).

6. For more information on the topic see, Vijay Gorantla et al., "Composite Tissue Allotransplantation (CTA): Current Status and Future Insights," *European Journal of Trauma* 6 (2001), 267–74.

7. Dr. L. Scott Levin at Duke University, for example, has transplanted a big toe onto a hand for use as an opposable thumb.

8. Simon Hattenstone, "Face Saver," *The Guardian*, November 10, 2007, http://www.guardian.co.uk/lifeandstyle/2007/nov/10/healthandwellbeing.features1.

9. W. Zimmerman, "Legend of the black leg, 348 AD." *One leg in the grave: the miracle of the transplantation of the black leg by the Saints Cosmas and Damian.* Maarseen, Amsterdam, Holland: Elsvier/Bunge, Maarssen, 1998.

10. In 2006, a Canadian team reported that they had transferred one leg from an ischiopagus (also known as conjoined) twin. While the procedure was successful and involved a lower extremity, because it was on a genetically identical twin, it is not really considered an allotransplantation and no immunosuppressant drugs

were administered. R. M. Zuker, Redett, R., Alman B. et al., "First Successful Lower-Extremity Transplantation: Technique and Functional Result," *Journal of Reconstructive Microsurgery* 22 (2006): 239–44.

11. Chad R. Gordon et al., "From Experimental Rat Hindlimb to Clinical Face Composite Tissue Allotransplantation: Historical Background and Current Status," *Microsurgery* 26 (2006): 566–72.

12. M. Birchall, "Tongue Transplantation," *The Lancet* 363 (2004): 1663.

13. George Monks (1853–1933), "Correction by Operation, of Some Nasal Deformities and Disfigurements," *Boston Medical and Surgical Journal* 139 (1988): 262. Reprinted in *Plastic and Reconstructive Surgery* 48, no. 5 (1971): 485-91.

14. Martha Teach Gnudi and Webster, Jerome Pierce, *The Life and Times of Gaspare Tagliacozzi Surgeon of Bologna* (New York: Herbert Reichner, 1950), 282.

15. For more on Murray see, Joseph E. Murray, *Surgery of the Soul: Reflections on a Curious Career* (Sagamore Beach, MA: Science History Publications/USA, 2001).

16. Bohdan Pomahac, personal interview, August 15, 2008.

17. R. Gilbert, "Transplant is Successful with a Cadaver Forearm," *Medical Tribune Medical News* 5 (1964): 20.

18. J. F. Borel et al., "Biological Effects of Cyclosporine A: A New Antilymphocytic Agent," *Inflammation Research* 43 (1994), 179–86.

19. No authors listed. "A Randomized Clinical Trial of Cyclosporine in Cadaveric Renal Transplantation. Analysis at three years. The Canadian Multicentre Transplant Study Group," *New England Journal of Medicine* 309 (1983): 809–15.

20. R. K. Daniel et al., "Tissue Transplants in Primates for Upper Extremity Reconstruction: A Preliminary Report," *Journal of Hand Surgery* [Am] 11 (1986): 1–8. I. Technical Aspects," *Plastic and Reconstructive Surgery* 89 (1992): 700–9.

21. G. B. Stark et al., "Hand Transplantation in Baboons," *Transplant Procedures* 19 (1987): 968–71.

22. Steven Hovius et al., "Allogeneic Transplantation of the Radial Side of the Hand in the Rhesus Monkey: I. Technical Aspects," *Plastic and Reconstructive Surgery* 89 (1992): 700–9.

23. K. Black and Hewitt, C. "Composite Tissue Transplantation Workshop," Washington, D.C.: Department of Veteran's Affairs, Rehabilitation Research and Development Service, 1991.

24. John Barker, Jones, J., and Breidenbach, W. "Composite Tissue Transplantation: A Clinical Reality?" *Transplant Procedures* [Invited editor] 30 (1998): 686–787.

25. John Barker et al., "Research and Events Leading to Facial Transplantation," *Replantation and Transplantation* 34 (2006): 238.

26. Lawrence K. Altman, "A Pioneering Transplant, and Now an Ethical Storm," *New York Times*, December 6, 2005, http://www.nytimes.com/2005/12/06/science/06prof.

27. Ibid.

28. Elizabeth Rosenthal, "Under a Microscope: High-Profile Cases Bring New Scrutiny to Science's Superstars," *New York Times*, December 24, 2005, http://www.nytimes.com/2005/12/24/science/24research.

29. Robert Walton and Levin, L. Scott, "Face Transplantation: The View From Duke University and the University of Chicago," *Southern Journal of Medicine* 99 (2006): 417–18.

30. Elizabeth Rosenthal, "Under a Microscope: High-Profile Cases Bring New Scrutiny to Science's Superstars."

31. Jean-Michel Dubernard et al., "Human Hand Allograft: Report on First 6 Months," *The Lancet* 353 (1999): 1315–20.

32. Lawrence K. Altman, "Doctors Who Transplanted Hand Ponder Their Surprising Patient," *New York Times*, October 6, 1998, http://query.nytimes.com/gst/fullpage.html?res=9A03E0D61E38F935A35753C1A96E958260&sec=&spon=&pagewanted=all.

33. Ibid.

34. Dubernard et al., "Human Hand Allograft: Report on First 6 Months," 1315–20.

35. Ibid.

36. Unfortunately a copy of the consent form for Clint Hallam could not be obtained.

37. Dubernard et al., "Human Hand Allograft: Report on First 6 Months," 1315–20.

38. Ibid., 1316.

39. Ibid.

40. Although it was reported in some print and electronic media that Clint Hallam's donor was killed in a motorcycle accident, it could not be confirmed for purposes here.

41. Dubernard et al., "Human Hand Allograft: Report on First 6 Months," 1316.

42. Ibid., 1316–17.

43. Lanzetta Marco et al., "Second Report (1998–2006) of the International Registry of Hand and Composite Tissue Transplantation," *Transplant Immunology* 18 (2007): 1–6.

44. Ibid.

45. http://www.google.com/imgres?imgurl=http://news.bbc.co.uk/olmedia/980000/images/_980069_clint_hallam_join150.jpg&imgrefurl=ht3Fq%3Dclint%2Bhallam%2Bimages&usg=_LCOTPnj55U37s71027MCvMVOVo4=&sa=X&oi=image_result&resnum=2&ct=im.

46. Dubernard et al., "Human Hand Allograft: Report on First 6 Months," 1315.

47. Ibid., 1319.

48. Altman, "Doctors Who Transplanted Hand Ponder Their Surprising Patient."

49. Weilie Hu et al., "A Preliminary Report of Penile Transplantation," *European Urology* 50 (2006): 851–53.

50. Gordon R. Tobin et al., "Transplantation of the Hand, Face and Composite Structures: Evolution and Current Status," *Replantation and Transplantation* 34 (2007): 277.

51. Michael Eigen, "The Significance of the Face," in *The Electrified Tightrope* (London: Karnac, 1993),

52. Francis Cooke Macgregor, "Facial Disfigurement: Problems and Management of Social Interaction and Implications for Mental Health," *Aesthetic Plastic Surgery* 14 (1990): 249–57.

53. Other substantial commentaries and exchanges on the ethics of face transplantation were published in the *Southern Medical Journal*.

54. Robert Farrer, "Psychological Considerations in Face Transplantation," *International Journal of Surgery* 2 (2004): 77–78.

55. For a helpful research article on the relationship between feeling and facial expressions, see Jessie VanSwearington et al., "Specific Impairment of Smiling Increases the Severity of Depressive Symptoms in Patients with Facial Neuromuscular Disorders," *Aesthetic Plastic Surgery* 23 (1999): 416–23.

56. Jonathan Cole, *About Face* (Cambridge, MA: MIT Press, 1998), 128.

57. Peter Bannister et al. "Mobius's Syndrome," *British Orthoptics Journal* 33 (1976): 69–77.

58. Jonathan Cole, *About Face*, 134.

59. Ibid., 140.

60. C. Y. Baker and L. H. Smith. "Facial Disfigurmenta and Personality," *Journal of the American Medical Association* 112 (1939): 301–4.

61. Erving Goffman, *Stigma: Notes on the Management of Spoiled Identity* (New York: Simon and Schuster, 1986).

62. I. Summerton and Agha, R. A. "Sociological Considerations in Face Transplantation," *International Journal of Surgery* 2 (2004): 82–83.

63. Vicky Houston and Bull, Ray. "Do People Avoid Sitting Next to Someone Who is Facially Disfigured?," *European Journal of Social Psychology* 24 (1994): 279–84.

64. Nichola Rumsey et al. "The Effect of Facial Disfigurement on the Proxemic Behavior of the General Public," *Journal of Applied Social Psychology* 12 (1982): 137.

65. Ray Bull and Stevens, J., "The Effects of Facial Disfigurement on Helping Behavior," *Italian Journal of Psychology* 8 (1981):111.

66. http://www.changingfaces.org.uk/Home.

67. Emma Robinson et al. "An Evaluation of the Impact of Social Interaction Skills Training for Facially Disfigured People," *British Journal of Plastic Surgery* 49 (1996): 281–89.

68. Craig S. Smith, "As a Face Transplant Heals, Flurries of Questions Arise," *New York Times* December 14, 2005, http://www.nytimes.com/2005/12/14/science/14face.html?pagewanted=print.

69. Nichola Rumsey, "Psychological Aspects of Face Transplantation: Read the Small Print Carefully," *American Journal of Bioethics* 4 (2004): 22.

70. Marcia K. Goin and Goin, John M., "Psychological Effects of Aesthetic Facial Surgery," *Advances in Psychosomatic Medicine* 15 (1986): 89.

71. Ibid., 90.

72. Ibid.

73. Ibid., 91.

74. Ibid., 93.

75. Laura Greenwald, *Heroes with a Thousand Faces: True Stories of People with Facial Deformities and Their Quest for Acceptance* (Cleveland: Cleveland Clinic Press, 2007).

76. Sander Gilman, *Making the Body Beautiful: A Cultural History of Aesthetic Surgery* (New Jersey: Princeton University Press, 1999).

77. Edgardo D. Carosella and Pradeu, Thomas, "Transplantation and Identity: A Dangerous Split?" *The Lancet* 183 (2006): 183–84.

78. Goin and Goin, "Psychological Effects of Aesthetic Facial Surgery," 84–108.

79. P. Morris and Bradley, A. et al., "Face Transplantation: A Review of the Technical, Immunological, Psychological and Clinical Issues with Recommendations for Good Practice," *Transplantation* 83 (2007): 115.

80. Allen L. Furr et al., "Psychosocial Implications of Disfigurement and the Future of Human Face," *Transplantation and Plastic Reconstructive Surgery* 120 (2007): 562.

81. Ruth La Ferla and Natasha Singer, "The Face of the Future," *New York Times*, December 15, 2005, http://www.nytimes.com/2005/12/15/fashion/thursdaystyles/15FACE.

82. Craig S. Smith, "As a Face Transplant Heals, Flurries of Questions Arise."

83. Ariane Bernard and Smith, Craig S., "French Face-Transplant Patient Tells of Her Ordeal," *New York Times*, February 7, 2006, http://www.nytimes.com/2006/02/07/international/europe/07face.html?_r=1&pagewanted=print&oref=slogin.

84. Benoit Lengele et al., "Facing up is an Act of Dignity: Lessons in Elegance Addressed to the Polemicists of the First Human Face Transplant," *Plastic Reconstructive Surgery* 120 (2007): 804.

85. Ibid.

86. Thanks to Jean-Michel Dubernard who provided the consent form for Isabelle Dinoire, trans. Alexandra Julio, 2008.

87. Working Party Report, "Facial Transplantation," *The Royal College of Surgeons of England*, (2nd Edition, 2006), 41.

88. N. Koss, Robson, M. C., and Krizek, T. J., "Scalping Injury," *Plastic and Reconstructive Surgery* 55 (1975): 439.

89. Graeme Miller, Anstee, John, and Shell, John A., "Successful Replantation of an Avulsed Scalp by Micro Vascular Anastomoses," *Plastic and Reconstructive Surgery* 58 (1976): 133.

90. Hui Jiang et al. "Composite Tissue Allograft Transplantation of Cephalocervical Skin Flap and Two Ears," *Plastic and Reconstructive Surgery* 111 (2005): 31e–35e.

91. Gilman, *Making the Body Beautiful: A Cultural History of Aesthetic Surgery.*

92. Ibid., 16.

93. Liz Kowalczyk, "Brigham's Doctors Will do Rare Face Transplants," *Boston Globe*, July 29, 2007, http://www.boston.com/news/local/articles/2007/07/29/brigham_doctors_will_do_rare_face_transplants.

94. Ariane Bernard and Smith, Craig S., "French Face-Transplant Patient Tells of Her Ordeal."

95. Bernard Devauchelle et al., "First Human Face Allograft: Early Report," *The Lancet,* 386 (2006): 203.

96. Ibid.

97. Peter E. Butler, Clarke, Alex, and Hettiaractchy, Shehan, "Facial Transplantation," *British Medical Journal* 331 (2005), 1349.

98. No author cited, "Face Transplant Patient Getting Back to Normal Life," *ABC News,* May 25, 2006, http://abcnews.go.com/Primetime/Health/Story?id=2001410&page=1.

99. Devauchelle et al., "First Human Face Allograft: Early Report," 204.

100. Ibid., 203.

101. Ibid., 205.

102. Ibid., 207.

103. Ibid., 205.

104. No author cited, "Face Transplant Patient Getting Back to Normal Life," *ABC News,* May 25, 2006, http://abcnews.go.com/Primetime/Health/Story?id=2001410&page=1.

105. Ronald C. Hamdy, "Face Transplantation: A Brave or Maverick Surgery?," *Southern Medical Journal* 99 (2006): 410–11.

106. Working Party Report, "Facial Transplantation," *The Royal College of Surgeons of England,* (2004), http://www.rcseng.ac.uk/rcseng/content/publications/docs/facial_transplant_report_2006.

107. Susan Okie, "Brave New Face," *The New England Journal of Medicine* 354 (2006): 890.

108. Thanks to Jean-Michel Dubernard for providing this informed consent document, trans. by Alexandra Julio, 2008.

109. Dubernard et al., "Outcomes 18 Months After the First Human Partial Face Transplantation," *The New England Journal of Medicine* 357 (2007): 2451–60.

110. Susan Okie, "Brave New Face," *The New England Journal of Medicine* 354 (2006): 889–94.

111. S. Guo et al., "Human Facial Allotransplantation: A 2-year Follow-up Study," *The Lancet* 372 (2008): 631–38.

112. http://ca.news.yahoo.com/s/afp/081220/health/china_health_science_transplant_1.

113. Laurent Lantieri et al., "Repair of the Lower and Middle Parts of the Face by Composite Tissue Allotransplantation in a Patient with Massive Plexiform Neurofibroma: A 1-Year Follow-Up Study," *The Lancet* 372 (2008): 639–45.

114. Dalibor Vasilic et al., "Risk Assessment of Immunosuppressive Therapy in Facial Transplantation," *Plastic Reconstructive Surgery* 120 (2007), 657–68.

115. Bodhan Pomahac, personal interview, March 2008.

116. Alessio Baccarani et al., "Technical and Anatomical Considerations of Face Harvest in Face Transplantation." *Annals of Plastic Surgery* 57 (2006): 483–88.

117. Maria Siemionow et al., "A Cadaver Study in Preparation for Facial Allo-graft Transplantation in Humans: Part II. Mock Facial Transplantation," *Plastic and Reconstructive Surgery* 117 (2006): 876-86.

118. Alessio Baccarani et al., "Technical and Anatomical Considerations of Face Harvest in Face Transplantation," *Annals of Plastic Surgery* 57 (2006): 483–88.

119. Maria Siemionow and Galip, Agaoglu, "Tissue Transplantation in Plastic Surgery," *Clinics in Plastic Surgery* 3 (2007): 351–69.

120. Michel Foucault, *The Birth of the Clinic* (New York: Vintage, 1994), 124.

121. Ibid., 16.

122. Ibid., 10.

123. Ray Kurzweil, *The Singularity Is Near* (New York: Penguin, 2006), 300–12. Although Kurzweil's brand of futurism claims to overcome many of the traditional humanistic prejudices that prevent a serious consideration of the body's material capacities, Kurzweil's privileging of intelligence is tantamount to a sort of technological animism that misses the centrality of the human body's individuation processes in the dynamic interaction that he refers to as "consciousness."

CHAPTER 2

1. Internet Movie Database. John Wayne Bobbitt biography, http://www.imdb.com/name/nm0001956/bio.

2. Ian Sample, "Man Rejects First Penis Transplant," *The Guardian*, September 18, 2006, 3, http://www.guardian.co.uk/science/2006/sep/18/medicineand health.china.

3. William Saletan, "Giving Head: The First Human Penis Transplant," Slate September 22, 2006, http://www.slate.com/id/2150153.

4. Michael Eigen, *The Psychoanalytic Mystic* (London: Free Association Books, 1998), 12.

5. Bill Hewitt, "Face Transplant Update: It Will Never Be Me," *People* July 23, 2007, 108.

6. Dan Newling and Barton, Fiona, "My Strange Life with Someone Else's Face," *PerthNow*, January 28, 2006, http://www.news.com.au/perthnow/story/0, 21598,17967407-950,00.

7. Craig S. Smith, "As a Face Transplant Heals, Flurries of Questions Arise," *New York Times*, December 14, 2005, http://www.nytimes.com/2005/12/14/science/14face.

8. Lawrence K. Altman, "At Arizona Conference, Praise for French Face Transplant Team," *New York Times*, January 19, 2006, http://www.nytimes.com/2006/01/19/national/19face.

9. Craig S. Smith, "Dire Wounds, a New Face, a Glimpse in a Mirror," *New York Times*, December 3, 2005, http://www.nytimes.com/2005/12/03/international/europe/03france.

10. Lawrence K. Altman, "French, in First, Use a Transplant to Repair a Face," *New York Times*, December 1, 2005, http://www.nytimes.com/2005/12/01/health/01face.

11. Lawrence K. Altman, "A Pioneering Transplant, and Now an Ethical Storm," *New York Times*, December 6, 2005, http://www.nytimes.com/2005/12/06/science/06prof.

12. Newling and Barton, "My Strange Life with Someone Else's Face."

13. Sarah-Kate Templeton, "Injured Troops Offered Faceswap," (2007): Timesonline.com, http://www.timesonline.co.uk/tol/news.

14. Smith, "As a Transplant Heals, Flurries of Questions Arise."

15. Ibid.

16. John Mack died on September 27, 2004, after being struck and killed by a car in London, England.

17. For a more detailed account of an alien abductee story, see Jim Sparks, *The Keepers* (Orem, UT: Granite Publishing, 2008).

18. It is interesting that, as gasoline prices are at their highest in U.S. history, military experts have made increasingly serious attempts to confess their beliefs in the presence of space alien encounters and subsequent government cover-ups.

19. Donald D. McNeil, Jr., "Insouciance Recaptured," *New York Times*, December 18, 2007, http://www.nytimes.com/2007/12/18/health/research/18face.

20. It is interesting that English face transplant surgeon Peter Butler has commented that although it is not the desired outcome, many people with highly distorted facial features would be fine with even a mask-like facial allograft. "But interestingly, when we've talked to patients about that, most people would say that I'd rather have a normal-looking mask than what I've got now." Simon Hattenstone, "Face Saver," *The Guardian*, Saturday November 10, 2007, http://www.guardian.co.uk/lifeandstyle/2007/nov/10/healthandwellbeing.features1.

21. No author cited, "Modern Day 'Elephant Man' Transformed by Full-face Transplant," (2008): *FOXNews.com*, http://www.foxnews.com/story/0,2933,340916,00.

22. For more information on the topic of facial symmetry, see Dahlia Zaidel et al., "Appearance of Beauty, Symmetry and Health in Human Faces," *Brain and Cognition* 57 (2005): 261–63.

23. Ruth La Ferla and Singer, Natasha, "The Face of the Future," *New York Times*, December, 15, 2005, http://www.nytimes.com/2005/12/15/fashion/thursdaystyles/15FACE.

24. Ibid.

25. Jon Bowen, "Gaining Face," (1999): Salon.com, http://www.salon.com/health/feature/1999/05/19/face_transplants.

26. John Litchfield, "Face Transplant Recipient Isabelle Dinoire Faces the World," (2006): *The Independent*, http://www.independent.co.uk.

27. Lawrence K. Altman, "At Arizona Conference, Praise for French Face Transplant Team," *New York Times*, January 19, 2006, http://www.nytimes.com/2006/01/19/national/19face.

28. Hattenstone, "Face Saver."

29. Or, to use the term Donna Haraway borrows from the philosopher of science Karen Barad, "intra-actions."

30. Donna J. Haraway, *When Species Meet* (Minneapolis: The University of Minnesota Press, 2008), 16.

31. Ibid., 15.

32. Ibid., 17.

33. Kate Franklin, "Tumour Sufferer Has Face Transplant," *Telegraph*, March 26, 2008, http://www.telegraph.co.uk/news/worldnews/1582576/Tumour-sufferer-has-face-transplant.

34. Ibid.

35. Haraway, *When Species Meet*, 16.

36. Bruce Wagner, *Memorial* (New York: Simon & Schuster, 2006), 80.

37. Celebrity gossip from Perez Hilton, http://perezhilton.com/category/knifestyles.

38. Grant Rollings, "I Only See Me in the Mirror," *The Sun*, November 27, 2006, http://www.thesun.co.uk/sol/homepage/news/article72845.ece/. *The Sun*, among other British tabloids, has shown a far greater interest in Dinoire's case than American tabloids have.

39. *Cracked*, "Playing God Never Looked So Good." December 17, 2007, http://www.cracked.com/blog/tag/face-transplant

CHAPTER 3

1. Christopher Lasch, *The Culture of Narcissism. American Life in an Age of Diminishing Expectations* (New York: Warner Books, 1979), 30.

2. Christopher Lasch, *Haven in a Heartless World: The Family Besieged* (New York: W. W. Norton and Co., 1995).

3. Heidi Murkoff, *What to Expect When You're Expecting*, 4th ed. (New York: Workman Publishing Company, 2008).

4. Lasch, *The Culture of Narcissism*, 38; Murkoff, *What to Expect When You're Expecting*.

5. Melanie Klein, "The Oedipus Complex in the Light of Early Anxieties" in *Contributions of Psychoanalysis* (New York: McGraw-Hill, 1964).

6. *Aliens*, directed by James Cameron (1986; Los Angeles, CA: Twentieth Century-Fox Film Corporation).

7. *The Matrix*, directed by Andy Wachowski and Larry Wachowski (1999; Burbank, CA: Groucho II Film Partnership/Warner Bros.).

8. *Everything You Always Wanted to Know About Sex* But Were Afraid to Ask*, directed by Woody Allen (1972; Hollywood, CA: Rollins-Joffe Productions).

9. Donald Winnicott, *Playing and Reality* (London: Tavistock), 111.

10. Ibid., 114.

11. Ibid., 112.

12. Edward Tronick et al., "The Infant's Response to Entrapment Between Contradictory Messages in Face-to-Face Interaction," *Journal of the American Academy of Child Psychiatry* 17 (1978), 1–13.

13. Winnicott, *Playing and Reality*, 113.

14. Lucy Grealy, *Autobiography of a Face* (New York: Houghton Mifflin), 111.

15. Peter Allen, "World's First Face Transplant Patient: My Horror of Sharing Body with Other Woman," October 2007, *Mail Online*, http://www.dailymail.co.uk/news/article-484998/Worlds-face-transplant-patient-My-horror-sharing-body-woman.

16. Ibid.

17. *WALL-E*, directed by Andrew Stanton (2008; Burbank, CA: Walt Disney Pictures).

18. *Supersize Me*, directed by Morton Spurlock (2004; The Con).

19. Anna Freud, *The Ego and the Mechanisms of Defense* (1936; London: Karnac Press Books, 1993).

20. Didier Anzieu, *The Skin Ego. A Psychoanalytic Approach to the Self*, trans. Chris Turner (New Haven: Yale University Press, 1989), 15.

21. Nina G. Jablonsky, *Skin, A Natural History* (Berkeley, CA: University of California Press, 2006), 16.

22. Jonathan Cole, *About Face* (Cambridge: MIT Press, 1998), 29.

23. Ibid., 33.

24. Ibid., 32.

25. Anzieu, *The Skin Ego,* 16.

26. For more information on skin adornment and mutilization see, Victoria Pitts, *In the Flesh: The Cultural Politics of Body Modification* (Basingstoke, Hampshire, UK: Palgrave Macmillan, 2003).

27. Anzieu, *The Skin Ego,* 40.

28. For more information on Freud's ideas on feelings of oceanic oneness see, Sigmund Freud, *The Future of an Illusion* (1927; New York: W. W. Norton & Company, 1989).

29. Margaret Mahler, Pine, Fred, and Bergman, Anni, *The Psychological Birth of the Human Infant: Symbiosis and Individuation* (New York: Basic Books, 1975).

30. Anzieu, *The Skin Ego.*

31. Adam Phillips, *On Kissing, Tickling and Being Bored* (Boston: Harvard University Press, 1998), 9.

32. Anzieu, *The Skin Ego*, 42.

33. *Dark Passage,* directed by Delmer Daves (1947; Burbank, CA: Warner Brothers Pictures).

34. Anzieu, *The Skin Ego*, 98.

35. Ibid., 99.

36. Anzieu, *The Skin Ego*, 102.

37. Ibid., 103.

38. Ibid.

39. Ibid., 106.

40. Ibid., 103.

41. Bill Hewitt, "Face Transplant Update: It Will Never Be Me," *People* July 23, 2007, 108.

42. Michael Eigen, *The Psychoanalytic Mystic* (London: Free Association Books, 1998).

43. Ibid., 21.

CHAPTER 4

1. Including photos that, current for the time, presented Dinoire beaming with elation in various poses counterbalanced against earlier grisly photographs of her before surgery.

2. Bill Hewitt, "Face Transplant Update: It Will Never Be Me," *People* July 23, 2007, 108.

3. Fox News, AP, December 13, 2007.

4. Hewitt, Ibid.

5. Ample examples of these contestations can be found in gender theory, epistemology, and psychological and biological development—the concerns of which are not at issue here.

6. Sigmund Freud, *Totem and Taboo*, trans. J. Strachey (New York: W.W. Norton & Co., 1962).

7. Ibid., 376.

8. Alexander Theroux, "Revenge," *Harper's* October, 1982, 27.

9. Sigmund Freud, "A Note upon the 'Mystic Writing-Pad.'" trans. J. Strachey, *International Journal of Psycho-Analysis* (1940): 469–74.

10. Ibid.

11. Ibid.

12. Ibid.

13. Bill Hewitt, "Face Transplant Update: It Will Never Be Me."

14. http://www.cindyjackson.

15. Jacques Lacan, *Ecrits*, trans. B. Fink (New York: W.W. Norton & Co., 2006).

16. Ibid.

17. Ibid.

18. Slavoj Zizek, *The Parallax View* (New York: Verso Press, 2006), 137.

19. The theme of crime and transplant procedures is interesting to ponder. For instance, interestingly enough, part of the large public outcry against the public release of the film in 1925 came from German police concerned over the fact that the film gave hints to audience members as to how to falsify one's fingerprints, an interesting fear that clearly has less to do with public safety than with what it might mean for a system of identity records used for the classification and recording of criminal identities. Perhaps when it comes to our pasts, we all feel a bit criminal.

20. Jean-Michel Dubernard, et al. "Human Hand Allograft: Report on First 6 Months," *Lancet* 353 (1999): 1316.

21. Roger Boyes, "Doctor's Hail Farmer's Double Arm Transplant," *The Times*, August 1, 2008.

22. Foreign Staff, "Pictures of 'World-first' Double Arm Transplant," *The Telegraph*, August 1, 2008.

23. Henri Bergson, *Creative Evolution,* trans. Arthur Mitchell (New York: Random House, 1944), 3.

CHAPTER 5

1. Roland Barthes, *Mythologies*, trans. A. Lavers (New York: Hill and Wang, 1972), 57.

2. Ibid.

3. Ibid.

4. Ibid.

5. Ibid.

6. Charles Tilly, *Why?* (Princeton: Princeton University Press, 2006), 65.

7. Mikhail Bakhtin, *Problems of Dostoevsky's Politics*, trans. C. Emerson (Minneapolis: University of Minnesota Press, 1984), 293.

8. Ibid., 128.

9. Ibid., 69.

10. Bill Zehme, *Lost In The Funhouse: The Life and Mind of Andy Kaufman* (New York: Delacorte Press, 1999), 198.

11. Ibid.

12. Viktor Shklovsky, *Energy of Delusion: A Book on Plot*, trans. S. Avagyan (Urbana-Champaign, IL: Dalkey Archive Press, 2007), 178.

13. Mikhail Bakhtin, *Rabelais and His World,* trans. Hélène Iswolsky (Bloomington, IN: Indiana Univeristy Press, 1984).

14. Gilles Deleuze and Guattari, Felix, *A Thousand Plateaus*, trans. B. Massumi (University of Minnesota Press, 1987), 170.

15. Ibid., 171.

16. Ibid., 181.

17. Ibid., 172.

18. Ibid., 190.

19. Ibid.

20. Dr. Bodhan Pomahac, personal interview, August 2008.

21. Alex Clarke and Butler, Peter, "Face Transplantation: Psychological Assessment and Preparation for Surgery," *Psychology Health and Medicine*, 9, no. 3 (2004), Informaworld, via Duquesne University, Gumberg Library, www.sites.duq.edu/library

22. Donald W. Winnicott, *Playing and Reality* (London: Routledge, 1997), 116.

23. Sarah-Kate Templeton, "Injured Troops Offered Faceswap," *The Times*, December 2, 2007, final edition.

24. Susan Okie, "Brave New Face," *The New England Journal of Medicine* 354, no. 9 (2006): 889–94.

25. Joan Didion, *The White Album* (New York: Washington Square Press, 1980), 11.

26. BBC News Online Network. From Hand to Face. September 20, 1998, http://news.bbc.co.uk/1/hi/health/183870.

CONCLUSION

1. S. Templeton, "Injured Troops Offered Faceswap" *The Sunday Times*, December 2, 2007.

2. Ibid.

3. Jeffrey Kluger, "Behind a Face Transplants Breakthrough," *Time Magazine*, December 17, 2007; http://www.TIME.com/TIME/health/article/0.8599.1867285. 00.html.

4. Craig Smith, "Pa. Doctors Ponder Face Transplant Issues," *The Pittsburgh Tribune Review*, December 2, 2005.

5. Caroline Alexander, "Rivaling Nature," *Smithsonian*, February 2007.

6. Johns Hopkins Medicine, "Surgeons Rebuild Iraq War Veterans Entire Nose Using His Own Body Parts," Media Relations and Public Affairs, May 14, 2007, http://www.hopkinsmedicine.org/Press_releases/2007/05_14_07.

7. E. A. Torriero, "Disfigured Soldiers Are War's Dark Face," *Chicago Tribune*, May 27, 2008.

8. Caroline Alexander, "Faces of War," *Smithsonian Magazine*, February 2007.

9. Ibid.

10. For more on this theme of exposure and the range and scope of weapons in military history, see Manuel Delanda, *War in the Age of Intelligent Machines* (New York: Zone Press, 1991).

11. Terri L. Weaver et al., "Appearance-Related Residual Injury, Posttraumatic Stress, and Body Image: Associations within a Sample of Female Victims of Intimate Partner Violence," *Journal of Traumatic Stress*, 20, no. 6 (2007): 999–1008.

12. Ellie Levine et al. "Quality of Life and Facial Trauma: Psychological and Body Image Effects," *Annals of Plastic Surgery* 54, no. 5 (2005): 502–10.

13. Jonathan Shay, *Achilles In Vietnam* (New York: Simon & Schuster, 2005).

14. Jonathan Shay, *Odysseus In America* (New York: Scribner, 2002).

15. Nina Berman, *Purple Hearts: Back from Iraq* (London: Trolley, 2004), 10.

16. Ibid.

17. Ibid., The soldier is referring to his prosthetic arm.

18. Berman, *Purple Hearts: Back from Iraq*.

19. Holland Cotter, "Words Unspoken Are Rendered on War's Faces," *The New York Times*, August 22, 2007.

20. Ibid.

21. Mark Greer, "A New Kind of War," *Monitor on Psychology*, 36, (2005): 40.

22. William M. Welch, "Trauma of Iraq War Haunting Thousands Returning Home," *USA Today*, February 28, 2005.

23. Ibid., 44.

24. As an aside, the idea of one's being able to prevent the stress and trauma of war is a bit like trying to use psychological assessment to find a person who was psychologically "fit" to receive a face transplant; both are equally absurd notions.

25. Albert A. Rizzo, et al. "An Immersive Virtual Reality Therapy Application for Iraq War Veterans with PTSD: From Training to Treatment," http://www. dtic.mil/cgi-bin/GetTRDoc?AD=ADA430298&Location+U2&doc+GetTRDoc. pdf. December 2004.

26. Daniel Coleman, "'Virtual Reality' Conquers Fear of Heights," *The New York Times*, June 21, 1995.

27. A. A. Rizzo et al., "An Immersive Virtual Reality Therapy Application for Iraq War Veterans with PTSD: From Training to Toy to Treatment."

28. Ibid.

29. Joann Difede and Hoffman, Hunter G., "Virtual Reality Exposure Therapy for World Trade Center Post-traumatic Stress Disorder: A Case Report," *CyberPsychology & Behavior*, 5 (2002): 529–35.

30. Hunter G. Hoffman, "Virtual Reality Therapy." *Scientific American*, August 2004, 60.

31. X. Jardin, *Virtual Reality Therapy for Combat Stress*, NPR. August 19, 2005, http://www.npr.org/templates/story/story.php?storyId=4806921

32. Amanda Schaffer, "Not a Game: Simulation to Lessen War Trauma," *The New York Times*, August 28, 2007.

Index

About the Authors

CARLA BLUHM is Developmental Psychologist and Visiting Assistant Professor at Allegheny College, in Pennsylvania. She has also been Assistant Professor or Adjunct Professor at Westminster College, University of Washington, Arizona State University, University of Rhode Island, and Columbia University.

NATHAN CLENDENIN is Doctoral Candidate in Clinical Psychology at Duquesne University. He has been an Instructor at Allegheny College.